Recent Advances in

Surgery

33

DATE DUE

GAYLORD		PRINTED IN U.S.A.

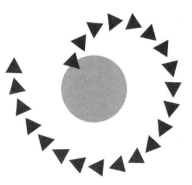

Recent Advances in

Surgery
33

Edited by

Colin D Johnson MChir FRCS

Reader and Consultant Surgeon, University Surgical Unit
Southampton General Hospital, Southampton, UK

Irving Taylor MD ChM FRCS FMedSci FHEA

Professor of Surgery, Director of Medical Studies and Vice Dean
UCL Medical School, University College London, UK

JAYPEE BROTHERS MEDICAL PUBLISHERS (P) LTD

New Delhi • St Louis (USA) • Panama City (Panama) • London (UK) • Ahmedabad
Bengaluru • Chennai • Hyderabad • Kochi • Kolkata • Lucknow • Mumbai • Nagpur

Published by
Jitendar P Vij
Jaypee Brothers Medical Publishers (P) Ltd

Corporate Office
4838/24 Ansari Road, Daryaganj, **New Delhi** - 110002, India, Phone: +91-11-43574357,
Fax: +91-11-43574314

Registered Office
B-3 EMCA House, 23/23B Ansari Road, Daryaganj, **New Delhi** - 110 002, India
Phones: +91-11-23272143, +91-11-23272703, +91-11-23282021, +91-11-23245672
Rel: +91-11-32558559, Fax: +91-11-23276490, +91-11-23245683
e-mail: jaypee@jaypeebrothers.com, Website: www.jaypeebrothers.com

Offices in India

• **Ahmedabad**, Phone: Rel: +91-79-32988717, e-mail: ahmedabad@jaypeebrothers.com

• **Bengaluru**, Phone: Rel: +91-80-32714073, e-mail: bangalore@jaypeebrothers.com

• **Chennai**, Phone: Rel: +91-44-32972089, e-mail: chennai@jaypeebrothers.com

• **Hyderabad**, Phone: Rel:+91-40-32940929, e-mail: hyderabad@jaypeebrothers.com

• **Kochi**, Phone: +91-484-2395740, e-mail: kochi@jaypeebrothers.com

• **Kolkata**, Phone: +91-33-22276415, e-mail: kolkata@jaypeebrothers.com

• **Lucknow**, Phone: +91-522-3040554, e-mail: lucknow@jaypeebrothers.com

• **Mumbai**, Phone: Rel: +91-22-32926896, e-mail: mumbai@jaypeebrothers.com

• **Nagpur**, Phone: Rel: +91-712-3245220, e-mail: nagpur@jaypeebrothers.com

Overseas Offices

• **North America Office, USA,** Ph: 001-636-6279734
  e-mail: jaypee@jaypeebrothers.com, anjulav@jaypeebrothers.com

• **Central America Office, Panama City, Panama**
  Ph: 001-507-317-0160, e-mail: cservice@jphmedical.com, Website: www.jphmedical.com

• **Europe Office, UK,** Ph: +44 (0) 2031708910, e-mail: info@jpmedpub.com

Recent Advances in Surgery 33

© 2010, Jaypee Brothers Medical Publishers

This book has been published in good faith that the material provided by contributors is
original. Every effort is made to ensure accuracy of material, but the publisher, printer and
editors will not be held responsible for any inadvertent error(s). In case of any dispute, all
legal matters are to be settled under Delhi jurisdiction only.

The cover of the book has been adapted with permission from the previous volumes published
by RSM Press (UK) for the title Recent Advances in Surgery.

Volume 33 First Edition: **2010**

ISBN 978-93-80704-22-7

Typeset at JPBMP typesetting unit
Printed at Sanat Printers, Kundli.

Contributors

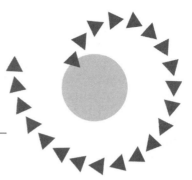

Shirish G Ambekar MBBS MS MCh DMS (Greenwich) FRCSEd(CTh)
Clinical Fellow, Department of Cardio-thoracic Surgery
Barts and The London NHS Trust, London, UK

Jonathan R Boyle MA MB ChB MD FRCSEd FRCSEng FRCS (Gen. Surg)
Cambridge Vascular Unit, Cambridge University Hospitals
Cambridge, UK

James P Byrne BSc (Hons) MD FRCS
Consultant Surgeon
Southampton University Hospitals NHS Trust, UK

Roderick TA Chalmers MD FRCSEd
Consultant Vascular Surgeon
Royal Infirmary of Edinburgh and University of Edinburgh, UK

RI Cutress PhD FRCS
Senior Lecturer and Consultant Surgeon, University of Southampton
and Southampton Breast Unit, Cancer Research UK Centre, Somers
Building, Mailpoint 824, Southampton General Hospital
Southampton, SO16 6YD, UK

Brian R Davidson MD FRCS
Professor of Surgery
Consultant HPB and Liver Transplant Surgery
Department of Surgery, Royal Free Campus
UCL Medical School, London, UK

Ziad El-Khatib MD
Endocrine, Bariatric and General Surgeon
Makassed Hospital, 11-6301 Beirut, Lebanon

Joanna Franks MBBS (Hons) BSc (Hons) MSc FRCS
Specialist Registrar in General Surgery
Division of Surgery and Interventional Science
University College, London, UK

Peter J Friend MA MB BChir FRCS MD
Professor of Transplantation, University of Oxford, UK

Kurinchi S Gurusamy MBBS MRCS MSc
Clinical Research Fellow/Honorary Clinical Teacher
Department of Surgery, Royal Free Campus
UCL Medical School, London, UK

Anil Hemandas FRCS
Specialist Registrar, Wessex Deanery, UK

Colin D Johnson MChir FRCS
Reader and Consultant Surgeon, University Surgical Unit
Southampton General Hospital, Southampton, UK

James Kirkby-Bott BSc MBBS FRCS (Gen Surg)
International Endocrine Surgery Fellow, Service de chirurgie
endocrinienne et général Hôpital Huriez, CHRU, Lille, 59037, France

Charles H Knowles BChir PhD FRCS (Gen Surg)
Senior Lecturer and Hon Consultant Colorectal Surgeon
Academic Surgical Unit, Centre for Digestive Diseases
Blizard Institute of Cell and Molecular Science
Barts and the London School of Medicine and Dentistry
Queen Mary University, London, UK

Sunil Kumar MS DNB FRCS (Ed) FRCS (Eng)
Senior Consultant and HOD Surgery
Tata Main Hospital, Jamshedpur, India

Peter J Lunniss MS FRCS
Clinical Senior Lecturer and Honorary Consultant Surgeon
Academic Surgical Unit, Centre for Digestive Diseases
Blizard Institute of Cell and Molecular Science
Barts and The London School of Medicine and Dentistry
Queen Mary University, London, UK

Patrick G Magee BSc MBBCh FRCSI FRCSEd FRCS(Eng)
Consultant Cardio-thoracic Surgeon
Department of Cardio-thoracic Surgery
Barts and The London NHS Trust, London, UK

Samir P Mehta MA DM FRCS
Clinical Fellow, Upper GI Surgery
Southampton University Hospitals, NHS Trust, UK

Isuru S Nammuni MBBS BSci (Med)
Specialty Registrar, Vascular Surgery Unit
Addenbrookes Hospital, Cambridge, UK

Karen P Nugent FRCS
Senior Lecturer in Surgery
University Surgical Unit, School of Medicine
Southampton General Hospital
Mailpoint 816, South Academic Block, Tremona Road
Southampton SO16 6YD, UK

Daniel O' Leary FRCSI FRCS (Gen)
Consultant Surgeon
Queen Alexandra Hospital, Portsmouth, UK

Amjad Parvaiz FRCS FRCS (Gen)
Consultant Surgeon
National Centre for Training in Laparoscopic Colorectal Surgery
Queen Alexandra Hospital, Southwick Road
Cosham Portsmouth PO6 3LY, UK

Sophie A Pilkington FRCS
Specialist Registrar, University Surgical Unit
School of Medicine, Southampton General Hospital, Mailpoint 816
South Academic Block, Tremona Road
Southampton SO16 6YD, UK

GT Royle MS FRCS
Consultant Surgeon, Southampton Breast Unit
Princess Anne Hospital, C Level, Mailpoint 132
Princess Anne Hospital, Southampton, SO16 5YA, UK

C Rubin FRCR
Consultant Radiologist, Southampton and Salisbury, Breast Screening
Unit, C Level, Mailpoint 132, Princess Anne Hospital
Southampton, SO16 5YA, UK

Michael A Silva MBBS MD MS FRCS (Gen) FRCS Ed
Consultant HPB Surgeon, Oxford Radcliffe NHS Trust, UK

Andrew L Tambyraja MD FRCSEd
Clinical Lecturer in Surgery
Royal Infirmary of Edinburgh and University of Edinburgh, UK

Irving Taylor MD ChM FRCS FMedSci FHEA
Professor of Surgery, Director of Medical Studies and Vice Dean
UCL Medical School, University College London, UK

Tim Underwood PhD MRCS
Clinical Lecturer in Surgery, Cancer Sciences Division
University of Southampton, UK

Arunima Verma MS
Department of Surgery, Tata Main Hospital, Jamshedpur, India

Preface

This latest volume of Recent Advances in Surgery 33 follows a familiar pattern. We have invited contributions, which address important and topical subjects in Surgery in General and in the major subspecialties of General Surgery.

In gastrointestinal surgery, we have chapters on pseudo-obstruction, pelvic floor disorders, therapeutic endoscopy and the surgical treatment of chronic pancreatitis and gallbladder cancer. Vascular surgery is moving forward into endovascular management but trauma is always with us and requires a range of traditional vascular surgical skills. Non-surgical advances have improved the results of treatment for breast cancer. We focus on the contribution made by the UK breast screening program.

As always, we take a wide-ranging look through randomized clinical trials and meta-analyses published last year, and we also have a contribution on the assessment of quality of trial publications, which we hope will be useful.

We are pleased to be working with our new publisher. We aim to maintain the high standards of the past, and we are confident that Jaypee Brothers Medical Publishers (P) Ltd., has produced a book of the highest quality, which will be valued by practicing surgeons and examination candidates in General Surgery.

Colin D Johnson
Irving Taylor

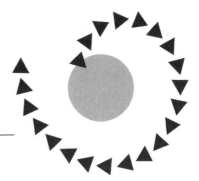

Contents

Section Five: Colorectal

Section Six: Vascular

Section Seven: Randomized Trials in Surgery

SECTION ONE

SURGERY IN GENERAL

CHAPTER ONE

Advances in Technologies in Operating Theaters

Shirish G Ambekar, Patrick G Magee

Surgery in its early days was limited to the drainage of abscesses, amputations of gangrenous limbs, extraction of decaying teeth and the treatment of trauma. Operations were carried out usually on kitchen tables in the candlelight by a person who had limited knowledge of the anatomy and physiology of the human body. Lack of anesthesia meant that they had to be performed swiftly without any consideration of asepsis, blood loss, analgesia or cosmesis. Mortality was high due to infections and shock. During the nineteenth and early part of the twentieth centuries, famous surgeons from the US and Western Europe performed surgery with an audience of medical students and even the general public. There would be a central table with galleries around it for the public to stand and watch. Hence, the name operating theater was coined (Figs 1.1 and 1.2).

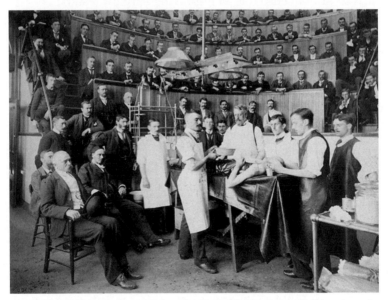

Fig. 1.1: Sir W MacCormac, a senior surgeon at St. Thomas' Hospital, London, about to perform an operation in Bellevue Hospital, New York in 1891 at the request of Prof Sayre (*Courtesy:* Wellcome Library, London).

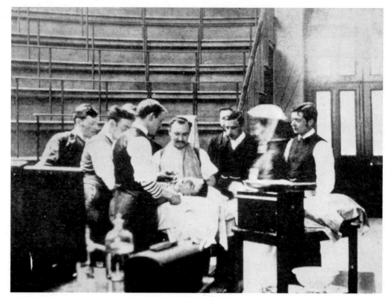

Fig. 1.2: An operation at St Bartholomew's Hospital, London. In 1910, the anesthetist, Charles Hadfield, is using a Vernon Harcourt apparatus (*Courtesy:* Wellcome Library, London).

In the last few decades various surgical specialties evolved. There was exponential growth in the knowledge and understanding of the working of the human body. Asepsis, antibiotics, anesthesia and transfusion services helped to reduce the mortality and morbidity due to surgery. Technology also played an immense role in improving surgical results.

Depending on the types of surgical work undertaken in the operating room (OR), the workload and the need for multiple specialties working together, different types of ORs can be built.

TYPES OF OPERATING ROOMS

Purpose Built Operating Rooms

Purpose built ORs for cardiac surgery, for example, will have space for cardiopulmonary support systems like a cardiopulmonary bypass machine, intra-aortic balloon pump and ventricular assist device. Those for gastrointestinal (GI) and urological surgery will need facilities for multiple scopes and monitors to display the operative field. Neurosurgery and ophthalmic ORs will have the facilities for operating microscopes, laser and magnetic resonance imaging (MRI).

Hybrid Operating Rooms

Hybrid ORs can facilitate the working together of different specialties at the same time and place. Interventional radiologists and vascular surgeons can perform stenting of aneurysms or injured vessels together and if the need arises, the patient can be operated upon in the same hybrid OR by the vascular surgeon. Cardiologist and cardiac surgeons can work in unison in such hybrid ORs and can perform various procedures like closure of congenital defects, percutaneous implantation of degenerated valves and angioplasty and bypass surgeries. Urologists and radiologists can treat conditions like renal stones with minimal access in the hybrid ORs with the facilities of C-arm, fluoroscopy and laser.

Mobile Operating Rooms

Mobile operating facilities can carry staff, OR and all other support systems that are needed to run such a service to an area, which may be remote from the permanent facility. Mobile ORs are very useful in battlefields (Fig. 1.3), remote villages in the developing world (Fig. 1.4) and also in

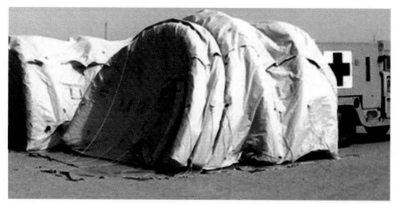

Fig. 1.3: Chemical and biological protective shelter, which can be inflated in 15 minutes and used as an operating room.[1]

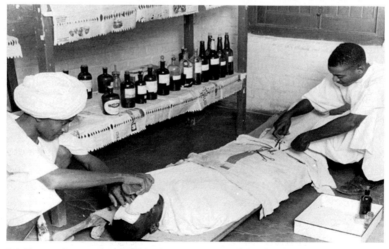

Fig. 1.4: Even today, surgical facilities in certain parts of the developing world are primitive and in such areas mobile ORs can make a big difference (*Courtesy:* Wellcome Library, London).

other situations, such as outer space or at sea. A large lorry, carrying a mobile OR, can go from place to place and doctors can perform basic surgical operations, and provide general health care services. In developing countries such mobile ORs can also be used for conducting camps for cataract removal, sterilization procedures, etc. In some countries, attempts have been made to use a cruise liner converted into a mobile OR facility that can be docked offshore. In this ultra modern facility, all sorts of major operations can be performed by highly trained staff coming from all over the world.

Modular Operating Rooms

Another new advance in operating theater technology is modular operating facility. Each module is built offsite and comes in packs, ready to be assembled on site. This module consists of a patient reception area, OR, anesthetic room, scrub area, sterile preparation room, equipment storage facility, laboratory, utility area or sluice, and changing and rest-rooms. These modules can be provided as a stand alone building that can be linked to an existing hospital or as a part of a multimodular facility that can be built for permanent or temporary use. These modular ORs are designed according to the needs of the health care provider and are built offsite. That means the site can be used for other purposes until the time of assembly. The time span from design to assembly can be as small as 10 weeks. Such modules can even be built from concrete where walls can withhold the weight of operating microscopes.

DIGITAL OPERATING TECHNOLOGY

Digital operating technology is the development of the last decade. It is mainly used in Minimally Invasive Surgery (MIS) viewing applications. A centralized control module routes images from numerous surgical and diagnostic imaging devices, for example, endoscopes, ultrasound, CT, MRI, fluoroscopy and patient monitoring data, within or across operative suites and these are then displayed to other departments, other hospitals or even overseas. Cutting-edge image acquisition technology used in modern cameras is used on overboard mounted optics to display real time high quality, wide-angled photographs and videos. Digital imaging technology enables ORs staff to control and manage all equipment and multiple imaging modalities and deliver the appropriate image in real time to the various specialists in the field. Integration of these different media with one cross-platform software, operating room media center (ORMC) was developed for the centralized control of all the surgical informatics systems.[2] Sterile touch screens provide effective barrier protection and prevent the transmission of microbial infections arising from contact with such instruments. Speech recognition software helps minimize the contact with the instruments. These digital technologies have enormous potential and can be a useful teaching and research tool where data can be stored electronically indefinitely. In future, when robotic surgery is likely to play a more important role, digital operating technologies are going to be the foundations of modern operating theaters.

The following points are to be taken into account during the planning and designing of a new OR facility:

- Maintain consistency of design with other ORs
- Avoid mirror image symmetry (Avoid people doing exactly opposite in one OR to that in another)
- Fire safety
- Accessibility (easy access to OR and the recovery room)
- Noise insulation
- Cleanability and maintainability
- Optimal use of space taking into account mobile and static equipment
- Safe power supply, lighting and supply of medical gases
- Facilities for data storage and data transfer (audiovisual streaming) for research, videoconferencing and telemedicine
- Facilities for the incorporation of robotic/minimal access surgery.

OPERATING THEATER EQUIPMENT

Each modern operating room is equipped with a set of high standard monitoring, diagnostic and digital equipment. The surgical side of the room has a pendant coming from ceiling, bearing a light source that is bright, shadow free and cold with a facility to either focus the light source or use it in a diffuse fashion (Fig. 1.5). Another pendant on the surgeon's side bears monitors, cameras and video equipment. There may also be another pendant for operating microscopes, but that may be wall mounted. Electrical diathermy (unipolar or bipolar) is usually placed at the foot end of the operating table. Modern diathermy machines are extremely safe and have built-in alarms to prevent patients getting burns in case of short circuiting of the electrical current. The operating table is operated electrically with a remote control that is placed on the anesthetist's side of the room. Modern tables can be tilted and folded in various angles and levels to give the surgeon optimal exposure (Fig. 1.6).

On the anesthetist's side of the room, there is a ceiling pendant that provides sources for piped medical gases, suction, electricity power supply and the supply of pressurized air for powering instruments, such as a surgical saw. On this side, there is also an anesthetic machine and other monitoring equipment. Basic monitors display electrocardiogram, arterial and central venous pressures, pulse oximetry and end-tidal CO_2. More sophisticated monitors can display pulmonary artery pressure, cardiac output, central core and peripheral temperatures, evoked motor or sensory potentials, electroencephalogram, cerebrospinal fluid (CSF)

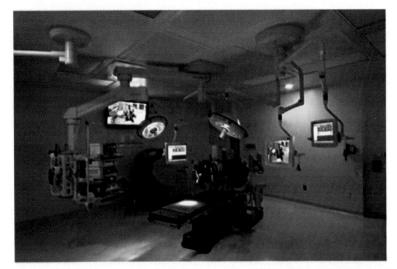

Fig. 1.5: Berchtold's supersuite combines bright, shadow-free CHROMOPHARE® lights, user-friendly TELETOM® equipment management systems and versatile OPERON® surgical tables to deliver the optimal surgical environment.[3]

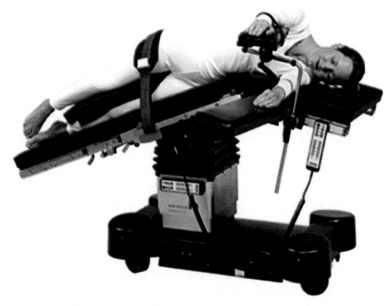

Fig. 1.6: OPERON® B 710—Surgical Table by Berchtold Corporation. When the patient is in the lateral position, the one-touch flex position provides excellent surgical site access during thoracic and kidney procedures.[3]

pressures, arterial blood gases and thromboelastograph (TEG) to assess coagulation. On the anesthetist's side, there is also a trolley for drugs and space to keep other relevant monitoring equipments like transesophageal echocardiogram (TOE), transcranial doppler (TCD) and multidrug syringe drivers that deliver various lifesaving medications, such as inotropes in accurate concentrations, calculated in micromoles per kilogram of patient's weight per minute.

Laminar Flow Ventilation

Laminar flow ventilation was first pioneered by Charnley in the 1960s and 1970s, for orthopedic operations like total hip and knee replacements. It resulted in a marked reduction in a postoperative deep-seated wound infection.

In a laminar flow ventilation technique ultra clean, bacteria free air is pumped into the operating room either in a horizontal or vertical fashion. The vertical method can be employed in an enclosed, semi-enclosed or open manner. While conventional or plenum type of ventilation maintains 20 air changes per hour, laminar flow ventilation can achieve 300 air changes per hour.[4] Colony forming units (CFU) are typically of the order of 150-300 cfus/m^3 in a conventional ventilation method while that number drops to less than 10 cfus/m^3 in the laminar flow method.[5] To be optimally effective, it is suggested that the operating room staff must wear body exhaust suits while working in this ultra clean environment.[6] These values were determined without considering whether prophylactic antibiotics were used or not, yet most experts feel that the use of antibiotics is the single most important factor in the reduction of the deep-seated infections. It was noted that by just increasing the air change rates there was no reduction in the clinical incidence of infections. More recent trials have tried to address this issue.[7, 8] Laminar flow ventilation is currently used widely in all modern operating theaters.

Cyberknife

Cyberknife is a new technology that is minimally invasive stereotactic robotic radiosurgery. Although it is not a conventional invasive surgical operation, it is a type of radiosurgery performed in specialized operative suits. It is used by oncologists and radiotherapists to treat deep-seated tumors in the body that were earlier thought to be untreatable due to the difficult access.[9,10]

With the use of robotic systems, multiple high resolution cameras and image-guidance high energy radiation beams can be delivered to the tumor with pinpoint accuracy. The "fall-off" of the radiation to the surrounding areas is rapid, giving protection to the healthy tissues (tissues that are 1 mm away from the tumor are protected). The Synchrony System is another software that can be used with the cyberknife to treat tumors that are in the vicinity of the chest and hence are moving with the respiratory cycle. A system of cameras, motion tracking software, fiber-optic sensing technology, infrared emitters and special tight-fitting elastic patient garments are used to track the motion of tumors and deliver the radiation accurately. This advance has revolutionized the treatment of many cancers and holds much promise for the future.

OPERATING ROOM OF THE FUTURE

Operating room of the future (ORF), a project pioneered by the Centre for Integration of Medicine and Innovative Technology (CIMIT), is currently running at Massachusetts General Hospital, Boston, USA. It is an OR with a conceptual design to try new technologies and new methods of anesthesia and operative workflow in a real setting. Its goals are:

a. To improve OR productivity by letting the operative and peri-anesthetic processes run in parallel rather than in sequence.
b. To improve the effectiveness of anesthesia personnel by creating a new, perioperative nursing position and including a self-contained recovery area in the unit.
c. To work near the limits of new technologies for the purpose of evaluating such equipment for more general deployment.[11] This project has also helped to track the response of all users in terms of emotional exhaustion and personal accomplishments and identify groups at high-risk for burnout when exposed to new systems and technologies.[12]

Experiences gained and the knowledge learnt from such innovative projects will help us push the boundaries of science and explore new frontiers in the fields of surgical technology, thereby enabling us to perform surgery in remote access areas, such as battlefields, outer space, at sea or even underwater.

REFERENCES

1. Peoples GE, Jezior JR, Shriver CD. Caring for the wounded in Iraq: A Photo Essay. New Engl J of Med 2004;351(24):2476-80.
2. Malarme P, Wickler D, Warzee N. Centralized control for surgical informatics systems in an integrated digital operating theatre. International Journal of Computer Assisted Radiology and Surgery 2008;3(Suppl 1):145-8.
3. www.berchtoldusa.com
4. Humphreys H. Infection control and the design of a new operating theatre suit. Journal of Hospital Infection 1993;23:61-70.
5. Lidwell OM, Lowbury EJL, Whyte W, Blowers R, Stanley SJ, Lowe D. Effect of ultra clean air in operating rooms on deep sepsis in the joint after total hip or knee replacement: a randomized study. British Medical Journal 1982; 285:10-4.
6. Hubble MJ, et al. Clothing in laminar-flow operating theatres. Journal of Hospital Infection 1996;32:1-7.
7. Van Griethuysen AJA, Spies-van Rooijen NH, Hoogenboom-Verdegaal AMM. Surveillance of wound infections and a new theatre: unexpected lack of improvement. Journal of Hospital Infection 1996;34:99-106.

8. Kelly AJ, Bailey R, Davies RG, Pearcy R, Winson IG. An audit of early wound infection after elective orthopaedic surgery. JR Coll Surg Edinb 1996;41:129-31.
9. Brown WT, Wu X, Fayad F, et al. Cyberknife radiosurgery for stage I lung cancer: results at 36 months. Clin Lung Cancer 2007;8(8):488-92.
10. Collins BT, Erickson K, Reichner CA, Collins SP, et al. Radical stereotactic radiosurgery with real-time tumor motion tracking in the treatment of small peripheral lung tumors. Radiat Oncol 2007;2:39.
11. www2.massgeneral.org/anesthesia/
12. Stahl JE, Sandberg WS, Rattner DW, et al. Introducing new technology into the operating room: measuring the impact on job performance and satisfaction. Surgery 2005;137(5):518-26.

SECTION TWO

BREAST

CHAPTER TWO

UK Breast Screening
After 20 Years

RI Cutress, C Rubin, GT Royle

INTRODUCTION

Breast cancer is the second most common cause of death from cancer in women in the United Kingdom (UK) after lung cancer. In 2006, more than 45,500 women were diagnosed with breast cancer and incidence rates have increased by over 50% in the last 25 years.[1] The risk of developing breast cancer increases with age and 8 out of 10 breast cancers are diagnosed in women over the age of 50 years. With the exception of certain high-risk groups, primary prevention of breast cancer is not currently a realistic strategy. In contrast, population screening represents an attractive option for reducing breast cancer mortality.

PRINCIPLES OF BREAST CANCER SCREENING

The classic criteria and principles of screening[2] are largely applicable to breast cancer screening by mammography. Breast cancer is a common disease with a recognizable and detectable early stage that can be satisfactorily treated. Current models of breast cancer biology recognize an early phase[3] where metastasis is less likely, and treatment is more likely to result in a favorable outcome. Furthermore, survival and other analysis by stage in early breast cancer and ductal carcinoma *in situ* (DCIS) detected within screening programs suggests this to be the case.[4,5] Such early disease is often detectable with reasonable accuracy by mammography, which has proven acceptable in various screening programs. The principle is that the screening test, in this case of mammography, sorts the population into positive and negative groups. It is important that as many people with the disease as possible are detected and the sensitivity for screening mammography from almost four million US screening mammograms has been reported at 81.2%.[6] It is also important that the number of people sorted in the positive group, who do not have the disease, is minimized and the specificity of screening mammography has been reported at 91.2%. Those sorted into the positive group then undergo appropriate diagnostic tests to determine if they do or do not have breast cancer. Overall risk benefit ratios and cost effectiveness will in addition also depend on program performance, hence, the importance of quality assurance, and this will be further discussed.

THE EVIDENCE FOR BREAST SCREENING

While mammography does fulfil many of the criteria required for a screening test simply comparing outcomes between cancers detected by screening and other means may not in itself provide evidence that screening can reduce breast cancer mortality. This is because of the various biases that may occur. Lead time bias occurs due to early detection of disease leading to an apparent increase in survival, when overall survival is unchanged but length of time with disease is increased due to earlier diagnosis. Length bias occurs due to preferential detection of slower growing tumors by screening because these tumors have a longer pre-symptomatic phase and are therefore more likely to be present during any given screening round. Faster growing tumors are more likely to present between screening rounds as interval cancers. Selection bias may occur when women who take-up the offer of screening differ from those who do not. For example, they may be more health conscious, have less comorbidity or come from differing socioeconomic groups. Randomized controlled trials aim to eliminate many of these biases and it is for these reasons that they produce important evidence as to the efficacy of screening.

The main randomized controlled trials comparing groups randomized to invitation to screening by mammography have been extensively reviewed[7] and summarized (Table 2.1). There have been criticisms leveled at some of the individual trials, for example, there are slight variations in age between the treatment and control groups in the Swedish two-county trial that has been interpreted to indicate flawed randomization processes, and the incidence of node positive disease was unexpectedly higher in the screened groups in the Canadian studies than in other studies and the control group with no obvious explanation. Additionally, contamination occurred in some studies where women in the unscreened group did in fact have screening out with the study. In summary, however, the Swedish Two-County trial overall produced a reduction in relative risk of 0.68 (95% CI: 0.59-0.80).[8] Other individual trials, while mostly demonstrating a trend towards risk reduction, were not always individually statistically significant (Table 2.1). It is for this reason that they have been combined in meta-analyses. Much of the controversy relates to which trials should be included and excluded from these meta-analyses given some of the criticisms described. The US preventive services task force meta-analysis excluded the Edinburgh trial and reported an overall risk of reduction for the remaining 7 trials of 0.81 (CI: 0.77-0.91).[9] In contrast, the Cochrane review by Olsen and Gotzsche only included two of the trials and reported a relative risk with screening mammography of 1.02 (95% CI: 0.95-1.10).[10] Overall, however, it is now generally accepted that these trials demonstrate

TABLE 2.1

Summary of randomized trials of breast screening with mammography[7,8]

Trial	Enrollment	Age	Population in thousands Screened: Control	Follow-up (mean duration)	Relative Risk (95% CI)
Health Insurance Plan, USA	1963-66	40-64	30:31	18	0.78 (0.61-1.00)
Malmo I, Sweden	1976-78	45-70	21:21	19.2	0.81 (0.66-1.00)
Malmo II, Sweden	1978-90	43-49	10:8	9.1	0.65 (0.39-1.08)
Kopparberg, Swedish Two-County	1976-78	40-74	28:18	20	0.59 (0.47-0.75)
Ostergotland, Swedish Two-County	1978-81	40-74	39:38	17.4	0.89 (0.72-1.09)
Edinburgh, UK	1978-81	45-64	29:26	12.6	0.78 (0.62-0.97)
Canadian I	1980-85	40-49	25:25	13	1.06 (0.80-1.40)
Canadian II	1980-85	50-59	20:20	13	1.02 (0.78-1.33)
Stockholm, Sweden	1981-83	40-64	39:21	14.9	0.90 (0.63-1.28)
Goteborg, Sweden	1982-84	40-59	21:29	13.3	0.78 (0.57-1.07)
UK Age	1991-97	39-48	54:107	10	0.83 (0.66-1.04)

a mortality reduction from breast cancer with screening mammography.[8,9] Finally, there are arguments as to whether breast cancer disease-specific mortality or overall mortality is the ideal endpoint for these trials. Overall mortality would enable inclusion of any unknown harms unrelated to breast cancer, but possibly related to breast cancer treatment or screening, in the risk benefit ratio. While on the surface this appears reasonable, none of the trials were powered to demonstrate a reduction in all cause mortality as such a study would need to be an order of magnitude larger than the trials conducted, since many of the women screened did not develop breast cancer. In fact, since the mortality from breast cancer is lower than many other cancer groups, many breast cancer trails use disease specific rather than all cause endpoints. Finally, in patients with breast cancer in the Swedish two-county trial, the overall mortality was reduced by screening.[11]

It has generally been accepted that the meta-analysis demonstrates a reduction in breast cancer mortality with screening and the debate has progressed onwards from criticisms of the internal validity of the various randomized controlled trials to questions of the external validity, or applicability of the trials of breast cancer screening to the real world.[12] Several studies have assessed the effectiveness of breast cancer screening programs. Interestingly, analyses comparing populations screened within screening programs with other control groups, such as historical controls suggests that in the real world the benefits of breast cancer screening with mammography are consistent with, and in some instances, in those screened, may even actually exceed the benefits seen in clinical trials.[13,14] Clearly, such non-randomized cohort studies may be vulnerable to the biases that the randomized trial aim to eliminate but there are several good reasons why outperformance of the trials by screening programs may be plausible. The trials compared groups by intention to screen and contamination of the groups by patients in the screening group not attending or patients in the control group attending screening would reduce the estimates of the benefit. Also current screening mammography equipment, machinery quality control and diagnostic skills have moved on from the time the trials were performed and would be expected to produce improved outcomes.

Key Point

- Meta-analyses of the randomized controlled trials and cohort studies suggest that screening by mammography reduces the mortality from breast cancer by 20-30%.

DEVELOPMENT OF THE NATIONAL HEALTH SERVICE BREAST SCREENING PROGRAM (NHSBSP)

Prior to the introduction of the national health service breast screening program (NHSBSP), the UK had the highest mortality rate from breast cancer in the world.[15] In response to this the Forest Committee was convened in 1985 and reported the following year.[16] In response to the recommendations, the world's first national breast screening program was set-up in England in 1988. Women, aged 50-64, were invited for single-view screening mammography. In 1995, the initial prevalent screen was increased to two views and this was subsequently rolled out to all screens in the NHS Cancer Plan 2000 in response to the United Kingdom Coordinating Committee on Cancer Research (UKCCCR) 2-view trial. The NHS cancer plan also called for age extension till 70. Further developments have included increased mammography film density,[17] double reading of mammograms[18] and better mammography equipment with higher resolution film. The screening interval has however remained constant at three years during the duration of the program. Future changes include further age extension by one screen at each end to increase the age from 47 to 73, the introduction of screening for those with a strong family history and gene mutation carriers and the replacement of analogue mammography equipment with full-field digital mammography. This was outlined in cancer reform strategy (CRS) to occur by 2012.

Controversy has often surrounded the age at which screening should occur. Breast density increases as those screened are younger and this effect is potentiated by the influence of hormone replacement therapy. The accuracy of mammography is therefore reduced and demonstration of benefit becomes less clear.[19] The randomized controlled trials on the whole were not designed or powered to demonstrate efficacy in differing age groups through subgroup analysis.[20] It does appear however that screening is of benefit in the age group of 40-50[9] although the trails took longer to longer to mature and find a difference in these groups. This is possibly because in a younger population, earlier lesions were identified and corresponding lesions took longer to develop in control groups than in older cohorts. Screening in patients older than 70 years of age under the NHSBSP occurs by self-referral only, as it was felt that there would be reduced uptake in this age group.

Key Points

- The NHSBSP screens women aged 50-70 with two-view mammography at three year intervals.
- This will be increased by one screening round at each end to ages 47-73 and will also include family history and high-risk screening and digital mammography, as outlined by the CRS to occur by 2012.

THE SCREENING PROCESS WITHIN THE NHSBSP

Following the detection of an abnormality at screening, women are recalled for assessment, which may include further views, ultrasound and clinical examinations. Possible radiological reasons for recall include the identification of a discrete lesion and asymmetry or microcalcifications. Histology is usually obtained either by ultrasound guidance or under stereotactic control if the abnormality is not seen on ultrasound. During the course of the NHSBSP, there has been reduction in the use of fine needle aspiration cytology (FNAC), which cannot distinguish between *in situ* and invasive cancer and may produce a higher rate of unsatisfactory aspirates in the presence of lobular carcinoma.[21] This has corresponded with an increase in the use of core biopsy and has helped reduce the open biopsy rate, for which there are quality standards and with the achievement of single stop targets.[22] Mathematical and other models have been developed to optimize the diagnostic yield following core biopsy.[23] Clinical examination is still an integral part of assessment following recall but is perhaps of more limited value in the presence of impalpable lesions. It is important however that any symptoms highlighted, such as nipple discharge or skin change, are properly assessed.

Introduction of breast screening has impacted on the presentation of breast cancer[24] with a consequent drive to improve the evidence base and management of smaller cancers and *in situ* disease. Surgery for impalpable disease includes the localization of any abnormality by ultrasound marking or with a guidewire.[25] Wires can be placed under ultrasound control or by mammographic control. Initially, under mammographic control wires had to be placed "freehand", which required considerable operator training. Stereotactic guidance is now widely used and has reduced operator dependence. Ultrasound marking of the tip of a wire placed under stereotactic control helps with surgical incision planning.[26] An alternative to wire placement is radioisotope occult lesion localization (ROLL), where radiolabeled technetium is injected into the lesion and a gamma counter used intraoperatively to enable localization in the same way that sentinel node biopsy is performed. This technique appears to be as effective as wire placement and may have advantages in some settings.[27]

Following specimen excision at surgery, the specimen is orientated with radiodense clips and the specimen is X-rayed to ensure the lesion is excised with adequate margins. Re-excision can take place under the same anesthetic if margins are close. Widespread specimen X-ray within the screening program has also lead to increased uptake of specimen X-ray within the symptomatic service and even with palpable lesions to better assess the adequacy of excision. Portable Faxitron machines in the operating theater have in some cases facilitated this and there do appear to be advantages to specimen x-raying of even palpable lesions.[28]

Key Points

- Breast screening has led to developments in and increased uptake of image-guided percutaneous biopsy techniques and image-guided surgery.
- Following ultrasound or wire-guided excision of impalpable breast cancer specimen orientation with radiodense clips and specimen radiography is important to assess adequacy of margins.

NHSBSP QUALITY ASSURANCE AND PERFORMANCE

In contrast to the treatment of symptomatic disease, screening takes asymptomatic women, many of whom have no symptoms or pathology, and subjects them to an intervention. Adequate quality assurance (QA) of the program is crucial to ensure that the risk benefit balance is favorable and has been embedded into the NHSBSP from inception. Reference centers for QA were established in 1989 and following identification of problems with the work of two radiologists in Exeter in 1997, QA was further tightened to ensure that the whole program operated to national standards. British Association of Surgical Oncology (BASO) and NHSBSP guidelines exist,[29,30] on all aspects of the screening and subsequent treatment process and were the first of their type for surgery in the UK and for screening worldwide. Rigorous attention to quality within the NHSBSP had a significant beneficial influence on symptomatic breast services within the UK and in part helped usher in one stop breast clinics for symptomatic patients.

As part of the screening process many aspects of the program's performance are audited and published as part of the NHSBSP and the

TABLE 2.2

NHSBSP selected program performance data.[31,32,39,40] The standardized detection ratio (SDR) is the ratio of the observed number of invasive cancers to the expected number. This is a key target indicator within the NHSBSP

Screening year	1996-97	2007-08
Radiological		
Number attending	1,558,995	1,994,651
Acceptance rate	75.2%	73%
Recall rate	66,333 (4.9%)	83,222 (4.2%)
Benign biopsy rate	3,268	1716
Invasive cancers < 15 mm	3,156	6,878
SDR (of those invited)	1.01	1.45
Surgical (Data are April to the following March)		
Number attending	1,340,175	2,042,497
Cancers detected	7410	16,792
	79% Invasive	79% Invasive
	20% *In situ*	21% *In situ*
	1% Unknown	
Mastectomy rate (invasive cancers)	27%	26%
Axillary nodal status (invasive cancers)	82%	98%
Radiotherapy rate after breast conserving surgery	Not recorded	92%
Repeat surgery	14.5%	20%
Preoperative diagnosis	62% (standard >70%)	95% (standard >85%)
Surgical caseload >20 screening cases PA	80%	92%
5 year survival	Diagnosis: 1990-91 93.6%	Diagnosis: 2001-02 97.2% (96.6-97.8)

Association of Breast Surgery (ABS) at BASO annual reports.[31,32] Examples of the types of data collected are illustrated in Table 2.2. The data from these reports has gradually demonstrated improved attainment of the various quality standards with time. Of particular note, the five years mortality has improved significantly during the program, and for NHSBSP patients with tumors that fall into the Nottingham Prognostic Index "excellent" and "good" prognostic groups, the survival is the same as for the general population.[32]

Key Point

- The NHSBSP is a quality-assured program and all aspects of diagnosis and treatment are audited against predetermined quality standards to ensure that the expected benefits are achieved.

AREAS OF CONTROVERSY

While it is now generally accepted that breast screening reduces mortality from breast cancer, arguments have moved on to operational issues and questions of the exact risk benefit ratio associated with breast screening. The randomized controlled trials have been criticized for including minimal data on the possible harms of breast screening and it is well documented that recall for further assessment causes a degree of psychological morbidity,[33] but that settles to baseline levels following the advice of a benign diagnosis. Some of the criticism has centered on the NHSBSP patient information leaflets, which it was previously felt by some aimed to persuade rather than discuss risk/benefit ratios. While not finalized, the NHSBSP patient information leaflets are now in the process of being changed and several papers have discussed the exact risk benefit balance in detail.[33] Central to this is that the information leaflets are in a format readily understandable to patients and figures, such as the numbers needed to screen to prevent one death from breast cancer are useful in this regard.[34] Estimates for this range from 465 using data from the Swedish two-county trial[34] to 1,224 obtained from a meta-analysis.[9] Further criticism relates to overtreatment, not only in terms of biopsies and diagnostic surgery for lesions that turn out to be benign but also of DCIS.[35] Incidence of DCIS has increased substantially since the introduction of screening programs and exceeds the levels of invasive cancers that would be expected indicating that at least some of the DCIS diagnosed through breast screening is not biologically relevant in that it would not have been expected to impact on the patient's life symptomatically in the absence of a screening program. Unfortunately, there is no way of knowing which DCIS may represent overdiagnosis and which is biologically important. It is therefore inevitable that there is some overtreatment but it is crucial that the overall risk benefit ratio is in favor of screening and that patient's consent to screening in an informed manner having had the opportunity to discuss these nuances.

> ## Key Point
>
> - For every 1,000 women screened for 10 years it has been estimated that three will avoid death from breast cancer. However, there is a 4 to 5% recall rate for further assessment at each screening round within the NHSBSP and some patients screened will be diagnosed with and treated for breast cancers that may have never become symptomatic.

FUTURE DEVELOPMENTS, RECOMMENDATIONS AND ADVANCES

Radiological

The NHSBSP has played an important role in recruitment of women to the Million Women Study, which demonstrated a link between the use of hormone replacement therapy and an increased incidence of breast cancer. The Sloane project, also recruited through the NHSBSP, is a prospective audit of screen detected noninvasive and atypical hyperplasias of the breast. The aim is to produce the largest such dataset of these conditions in the world.

Other important breast screening studies, which have led to changes in recommendations within the NHSBSP include the digital mammography imaging screening trial (DMIST)[36] performed in the USA, which demonstrated that while overall sensitivity between traditional screening mammography and digital mammography was similar, digital mammography performed better in younger women or women with denser breasts. The magnetic resonance imaging for breast screening (MARIBS) trial demonstrated that in women, aged 35–49, with a strong family history of breast cancer and a high probability of tumor protein p53 (TP53) gene mutation, contrast-enhanced MRI was of greater sensitivity than mammography for screening, and that a combination of the two detect the most tumors. The National Institute for Health and Clinical Excellence (NICE) Family History Guidance (CG41), which is due to be implemented through the NHSBSP, includes both modalities for these patients. For those aged 40-49 with a moderate family history of breast cancer, the FH01 study aims to assess the impact of mammographic screening on breast cancer mortality and results are awaited.

Surgical

Since breast screening leads to the detection of smaller cancers with less likelihood of nodal metastasis reduction of morbidity from axillary surgery is important. Surgical advances include the increased uptake of sentinel node biopsy. NICE guidance (CG80) recommends the staging of the axilla preoperatively with ultrasound, which will detect involved nodes in approximately two thirds of cases.[37] Fine needle aspirate of suspicious axillary nodes should reduce the false negative rate and these recommendations have been incorporated into the breast screening work up of newly diagnosed cancers prior to sentinel node biopsy in many units. Further advances will relate to intraoperative sentinel node analysis by molecular techniques, which have attained very high accuracy in described reports.[38] This will enable "one stop" axillary surgery avoiding the morbidity of axillary clearance in node negative patients and enabling node positive patients to avoid the delays, inconvenience and hazards of a second operation. Developments and increased uptake of oncoplastic and reconstructive surgical techniques have been evident in the treatment of patients with screen-detected disease. For example, the UK National Mastectomy and Reconstruction (MBR) audit demonstrates an increased uptake of immediate reconstruction from 11% nationally to 21% over the course of the study. It is of particular note that it is in those patients with widespread DCIS and therefore more likely to be screen-detected, the immediate reconstruction rate was 38%.

Key Point

- Sentinel node biopsy, including intraoperative sentinel node analysis and breast reconstructive and oncoplastic techniques reduce the morbidity and cosmetic sequelae of breast surgery.

CONCLUSION

In the last 21 years, breast cancer screening has been firmly established as part of the health care system within UK. It is generally accepted that screening does reduce the mortality from breast cancer but the risks and benefits should be clearly and honestly explained to women who then must decide whether to attend. Since benefit depends on the quality of the service and there is a risk of causing harm to women with no pathology, quality assurance procedures are crucial and have lead to improvements in both the standards of treatment of symptomatic disease and ensured a high quality of care for those within the program.

REFERENCES

1. Cancer Research UK Cancer Stats. Available at: http://info.cancerresearchuk. org/cancerstats/types/breast/index.htm.
2. Wilson JMG, Jungner G. Principles and practice of screening for disease. Bulletin of the World Health Organisation Volume 86, 1968. http://www.who.int/bulletin/volumes/86.
3. Hellman S. Karnofsky Memorial Lecture. Natural history of small breast cancers. Journal of Clinical Oncology 1994;12(10):2229-34.
4. Berry DA, Cronin KA, Plevritis SK, Fryback DG, Clarke L, Zelen M, et al. Effect of screening and adjuvant therapy on mortality from breast cancer. New England Journal of Medicine 2005;353(17):1784-92.
5. Wishart GC, Greenberg DC, Britton PD, Chou P, Brown CH, Purushotham AD, et al. Screen-detected vs symptomatic breast cancer: is improved survival due to stage migration alone? British Journal of Cancer 2008;98(11): 1741-4.
6. Breast Cancer Surveillance consortium performance measures for 3,884,059 screening mammography examinations from 1996 to 2007 by age. Available at: http://breastscreening.cancer.gov/data/performance/screening/perf_age.html.
7. Harris JR, Lippman ME, Morrow M, Kent Osbourne C. Diseases of the Breast. Chapter 11 ISBN978-0-7817-9117-5, 2009;87-116.
8. IARC Handbooks of Cancer Prevention. Volume 7: Breast Cancer Screening 2002. Available at: http://www.iarc.fr/en/publications/pdfsonline/prev/handbook7/index.php.
9. Humphrey LL, Helfand M, Chan BK, Woolf SH. Breast cancer screening: a summary of the evidence for the US Preventive Services Task Force. Annals of Internal Medicine 2002;137(5 Part 1):347-60.
10. Olsen O, Gotzsche PC. Cochrane review on screening for breast cancer with mammography. Lancet 2001;358(9290):1340-2.
11. Tabar L, Duffy SW, Yen MF, Warwick J, Vitak B, Chen HH, et al. All-cause mortality among breast cancer patients in a screening trial: support for

breast cancer mortality as an endpoint. Journal of Medical Screening 2002;9(4):159-62.

12. Harris R. Effectiveness: the next question for breast cancer screening. Journal of the National Cancer Institute 2005;97(14):1021-3.

13. Duffy SW, Tabar L, Chen HH, Holmqvist M, Yen MF, Abdsalah S, et al. The impact of organized mammography service screening on breast carcinoma mortality in seven Swedish counties. Cancer 2002;95(3):458-69.

14. Gabe R, Duffy SW. Evaluation of service screening mammography in practice: the impact on breast cancer mortality. Annals of Oncology 2005; 16(Suppl 2 ii):153-62.

15. The Forrest Report. Available at: www.cancerscreening.nhs.uk/ breastscreen/publications/forrest-report.html.

16. Wald NJ, Murphy P, Major P, Parkes C, Townsend J, Frost C. UKCCCR multicenter randomized controlled trial of one- and two-view mammography in breast cancer screening. BMJ 1995;311(7014):1189-93.

17. Young KC, Wallis MG, Ramsdale ML. Mammographic film density and detection of small breast cancers. Clinical Radiology 1994;49(7):461-5.

18. Brown J, Bryan S, Warren R. Mammography screening: an incremental cost effectiveness analysis of double versus single reading of mammograms. BMJ 1996;312(7034):809-12.

19. Berry DA. Benefits and risks of screening mammography for women in their forties: a statistical appraisal. Journal of the National Cancer Institute 1998;90(19):1431-9.

20. Fletcher SW, Black W, Harris R, Rimer BK, Shapiro S. Report of the International Workshop on Screening for Breast Cancer. Journal of the National Cancer Institute 1993;85(20):1644-56.

21. Patel JJ, Gartell PC, Smallwood JA, Herbert A, Royle G, Buchanan R, et al. Fine needle aspiration cytology of breast masses: an evaluation of its accuracy and reasons for diagnostic failure. Annals of the Royal College of Surgeons of England 1987;69(4):156-9.

22. Ibrahim AE, Bateman AC, Theaker JM, Low JL, Addis B, Tidbury P, et al. The role and histological classification of needle core biopsy in comparison with fine needle aspiration cytology in the preoperative assessment of impalpable breast lesions. Journal of Clinical Pathology 2001;54(2):121-5.

23. Coombs NJ, Laddie JR, Royle GT, Rubin CM, Briley MS. Improving the sensitivity of stereotactic core biopsy to diagnose ductal carcinoma *in situ* of the breast: a mathematical model. British Journal of Radiology 2001; 74(878):123-6.

24. Moody C, Corder A, Mullee MA, Guyer P, Rubin C, Cross M, et al. The impact of the first 3 years of breast cancer screening on the overall presentation of breast cancer. Journal of the Royal Society of Medicine 1994;87(5):259-62.

25. Campbell ID, Royle GT, Coddington R, Theaker J, Rubin CM, Guyer PB, et al. Technique and results of localization biopsy in a breast screening programme. British Journal of Surgery 1991;78(9):1113-5.

26. Kolpattil S, Crotch-Harvey M. Improved accuracy of wire-guided breast surgery with supplementary ultrasound. European Journal of Radiology 2006;60(3):414-7.

27. Rampaul RS, Bagnall M, Burrell H, Pinder SE, Evans AJ, Macmillan RD. Randomized clinical trial comparing radioisotope occult lesion localization and wire-guided excision for biopsy of occult breast lesions. British Journal of Surgery 2004;91(12):1575-7.

28. May D, Richardson C, Cutress R, Agrawal A, Yiangou C, Wise M. The effect of faxitron intraoperative specimen radiography on the management of palpable breast cancer within a single unit. British Journal of Surgery 2008;95[S3]:50-51.

29. Association of Breast Surgery at BASO. Surgical guidelines for the management of breast cancer. European Journal of Surgical Oncology 2009;35(Suppl 1):1-22.

30. Sibbering M, Watkins R, Winstanley J, Patnick J. Quality Assurance Guidelines for Surgeons in Breast Cancer Screening. NHSBSP Publication No 20, 2009. Available at: http://www.baso.org/content/Abs-Guidelines.asp.

31. NHS Breast Screening Programme Annual Review 2009. Available at: http://www.cancerscreening.nhs.uk/breastscreen/publications/index.html.

32. NHS Breast Screening Programme and Association of Breast Surgery at BASO. An audit of screen detected breast cancers for the year of screening April 2007 to March 2008. Available at: http://www.wmpho. org.uk/wmciu/PublicationSearch3LevelList.asp?Level=2andID=17.

33. Schwartz LM, Woloshin S. Participation in mammography screening. BMJ 2007;335(7623):731-2.

34. Tabar L, Vitak B, Yen MF, Chen HH, Smith RA, Duffy SW. Number needed to screen: lives saved over 20 years of follow-up in mammographic screening. Journal of Medical Screening 2004;11(3):126-9.

35. Jorgensen KJ, Gotzsche PC. Overdiagnosis in publicly organised mammography screening programmes: systematic review of incidence trends. BMJ 2009;339:b2587.

36. Pisano ED, Gatsonis C, Hendrick E, Yaffe M, Baum JK, Acharyya S, et al. Diagnostic performance of digital versus film mammography for breast-cancer screening. New England Journal of Medicine 2005;353(17):1773-83.

37. Tate JJ, Lewis V, Archer T, Guyer PG, Royle GT, Taylor I. Ultrasound detection of axillary lymph node metastases in breast cancer. European Journal of Surgical Oncology 1989;15(2):139-41.

38. Martin M, Veys I, Majjaj S, Lespagnard L, Schobbens JC, Rouas G, et al. Clinical validation of a molecular assay for intra-operative detection of metastases in breast sentinel lymph nodes. European Journal of Surgical Oncology 2009;35(4):387-92.

39. NHS Breast Screening Programme Annual Review 1999. Available at: http://www.cancerscreening.nhs.uk/breastscreen/publications/archive. html#annual-reviews.

40. NHS Breast Screening Programme and British Association of Surgical Oncology. An audit of screen detected breast cancers for the year of screening April 1996 to March 1997. Available at: http://www.wmpho. org.uk/wmciu/PublicationSearch3LevelList.asp?Level=2andID=17.

SECTION THREE

ENDOCRINE

CHAPTER THREE

Recent Advances in Parathyroid Surgery

James Kirkby-Bott, Ziad El-Khatib

This chapter concentrates on recent changes in our understanding of parathyroid disease and technology, their affect on parathyroid surgery and the ways surgical techniques have contributed to the success of minimally invasive approaches.

VITAMIN D DEFICIENCY AND PRIMARY HYPERPARATHYROIDISM (HPT)

The importance of vitamin D to endocrine surgery is increasing all the time. Abnormal vitamin D metabolism is responsible for secondary hyperparathyroidism (HPT) in the normal, as well as the renal population. In Northern Europe, vitamin D deficiency affects 25 to 50% of the population. In an era of increasing interest in surgery for mild and asymptomatic primary HPT, the measurement of vitamin D is essential to ensure the implementation of correct diagnosis as it causes parathyroid hyperplasia. To help in carrying out the diagnosis in patients with hypercalcemia, measurement of the ratio of calcium excretion to renal function can be diagnostic (Fig. 3.1). If the ratio is > 0.01 in the context of hypercalcemia and HPT, then primary HPT is certain. However, when the ratio is < 0.01 either another cause of hypercalcemia, such as familial hypocalciuric hypercalcemia (FHH) or Paget's disease is present; or vitamin D deficiency is suppressing the ratio in the presence of primary HPT.

$$\frac{(\text{Urine calcium (mmol/l)} \times \text{plasma creatinine (umol/l)}/1000)}{\text{plasma calcium (mmol/l)} \times \text{urine creatinine (mmol/l)}}$$

To convert mg/dl to mmol/l multiply by 0.25

Fig. 3.1: Formula for calculating whether plasma and urine calcium results equate to primary HPT.

Key Point

• When vitamin D deficiency is present, it should be corrected and the tests repeated.

Vitamin D deficiency has been associated with increased tracer uptake in methoxyisobutyl isonitrile stress (MIBI) scintigraphy, improving the sensitivity of this test in patients who have hypovitaminosis D and a primary parathyroid adenoma.[1] In addition, vitamin D has been shown to be associated with the late onset of hypocalcemia, one week after minimally invasive parathyroidectomy. The vitamin D deficient group also had lower serum calcium, 24 hours after surgery than the normal vitamin D group.[1,2]

GENE TESTING IN THE YOUNG

The prevalence of sporadic HPT in the young is also topical. Two large series[3] (Kirkby-Bott et al unpublished) both looking at cohorts of > 1,100 parathyroid operations noted that 5% of those under 40 years old had either a family history of HPT or a previously unknown positive gene test for the multiple endocrine neoplasia (MEN) 1 or 2 gene. Familial isolated HPT has been associated with HPT type 2 (HRPT2) gene mutations and this mutation is strongly linked with sporadic parathyroid cancer, but not with sporadic benign primary HPT.[4] Familial hyperparathyroid disease can be either multiglandular or adenomatous. In familial cases where the index case had adenomatous disease treated without recurrence, a focused approach is not contraindicated, but is in familial multigland disease. Either nonfamilial sporadic disease does occur in those under 40 years old or the responsible genes are yet to be found. The cure rate in the persons under 40 years of age without a family history or positive gene tests is comparable to the rest of the sporadic hyperparathyroid population suggesting that this cohort represents the tail end of one side of a normally distributed population suffering from sporadic parathyroid adenomas and they all do not have a multiple gland disease syndrome.

Key Point

- While many clinicians routinely refer patients under the age of 30 years for gene testing, expecting to detect a small number of genetic syndromes, there is no evidence at present to support this practice.

LITHIUM ASSOCIATED HPT

Lithium is associated with parathyroid hyperplasia and primary HPT.[5] This has been shown to be due to an alteration in the calcium sensing receptor, so that a higher serum calcium level is needed to trigger cellular pathways. Bone mineral density is not affected,[6] and there is no hypercalciuria that would predispose to nephrocalcinosis and renal lithiasis. During the diagnostic work-up for lithium-induced HPT, urine calcium measurements are usually normal. A review of 1207 primary HPT operations revealed 1.3%

were for lithium associated HPT.[7] It is not possible to calculate whether there is an excess risk of primary (adenomatous) HPT in those taking lithium compared to the general population. It may be that the few reports of adenomatous HPT, in those taking lithium, represent concomitant pathology unrelated to lithium-associated parathyroid hyperplasia, which does not require surgical treatment.

Key Point

- Surgery for lithium-induced HPT should be restricted to those with adenomatous disease diagnosed by concordant preoperative imaging.

INTRAOPERATIVE ADJUNCTS TO PARATHYROID SURGERY

The challenges facing the parathyroid include the identification of parathyroid tissue, ensuring the removal of all the diseased parathyroid tissue. There are many techniques that have been developed to help the surgeon confirm that he has found parathyroid tissue, including frozen section, IV methylene blue dye, radioguided parathyroidectomy (RGP) and tissue aspirate parathyroid hormone (PTH) assays. RGP works by giving the patient a radiolabeled tracer of the same compound given for SESTAMIBI scintigraphy (SESTAMIBI). A gamma probe then detects emitted gamma radiation from the labeled tracer to help pinpoint the gland. A positive preoperative SESTAMIBI is essential for this technique to be used.

Key Point

- Methylene blue cannot be recommended because of the risk of toxic encephalopathy.

A recent review paper has compared intraoperative adjuncts in parathyroid surgery.[8] Table 3.1 summarizes this paper with the addition of search results for tissue aspirate PTH.[9-11]

Key Point

- Harrison et al recommends using intraoperative PTH to confirm adequate resection in patients with disease localized by SESTAMIBI, but not for those with concordant SESTAMIBI and ultrasound (USS) results where it is of no proven benefit.

A developing technique using intraoperative tissue aspirates for PTH levels has been described in three papers. In the largest series (a prospective case-controlled trial), the technique had a sensitivity of 97%

TABLE 3.1

Comparing intraoperative adjuncts and the level of evidence for each.

Intraoperative adjunct	Level of evidence	Additional notes
Radioguided parathyroidectomy	Level IV, Grade C	Requires a positive preoperative MIBI scan.
Frozen section	Level III-IV, Grades B-C	Microscopic follicular variants can cause false negatives and positives.
Methylene blue	Level IV, Grade C	Risk of toxic encephalopathy especially if taking an SSRI drug.
Tissue aspirate PTH	Level IIb, Grade B	Few studies, not a well established technique, only validated in primary HPT.

and a specificity of 100%.[9] The false negatives are due to inadequate sampling and this is a recognized problem of the technique. In an ongoing study of this technique in Lille, France, samples that are considered to be inadequate by the operator are repeated with a success rate of 100% and the technique used is described in the press.[9,11] The current literature only reports this technique about primary HPT.

This technique may also have a role in familial hyperplastic disease and secondary hyperparathyroid disease. In subtotal parathyroidectomy, it is essential to confirm that the remnant being left is parathyroid tissue and any portion being sent for cryopreservation is also parathyroid. Therefore, the technique is invaluable as there are no reports of false positive results. Although frozen section has been shown to have an accuracy of 99.2%,[12] other papers report on the occasional inaccuracies of frozen section, including false positives and a failure rate of 2.5%.[13]

Key Point

- Tissue aspirates also have the advantage of no biopsy being required and multiple samples can be taken to help identify ectopic tissue and differentiate thyroid nodules and lymph nodes, without overburdening the histopathologists or risking permanent hypoparathyroidism.

CERVICOSCOPY

Advances in the accuracy of preoperative and perioperative localizing techniques have led to a preference for a minimally invasive procedure over bilateral exploration in image localized sporadic primary HPT. The focused approach has been shown to be equivalent to bilateral exploration for cure rate and superior to it concerning cosmetic result, duration of the intervention, postoperative stay and hypocalcemia as assessed by

TABLE 3.2

Comparison of techniques for cervicoscopy

	Endoscopic parathyroidectomy by Gagner	Video-assisted parathyroidectomy by Henry	Minimally invasive video-assisted parathyroidectomy by Miccoli
Number of trocars	3-4	3	0
Endoscope	5 mm	10 mm	5 mm
Endoscope angle	Initial 0°, then 30°	0°	30°
Other trocars	3-5 mm	2.5 mm	-
CO_2 insufflation	10 mm Hg	8 mm Hg	No
Bilateral approach	No	No	Yes

prospective and randomized trials.[14,15] During the last decade, multiple minimally invasive approaches have been described.[16] These include minimally invasive open parathyroidectomy, endoscopic and video-assisted parathyroidectomy and extracervical access from incisions in the chest wall and/or axilla.

The first endoscopic parathyroidectomy was described by Gagner in 1996. Minimally invasive video-assisted parathyroidectomy (MIVAP) was first described by Miccoli et al[17] and totally endoscopic parathyroidectomy (first described as video-assisted) by the lateral approach by Henry et al.[18] Currently, the best indication for this approach is adenomas that lie deep in the thyroid lobe, usually arising from superior gland adenomas. The video-assisted technique, first described by Miccoli, is a gas-less approach performed through a 1.5 cm midline incision located between the cricoid cartilage and the sternal notch. This technique has the advantage of a bilateral exploration from the same incision in case of suspicion of multi-glandular disease or inadequate preoperative localization studies.[19] Endoscopic parathyroidectomy by the lateral approach, described by Henry et al, is performed using carbon dioxide insufflation and a 12-mm skin incision on the anterior border of the sternocleidomastoid muscle, 3–4 cm above the sternal notch on the side of the affected gland. Prevertebral fascia is reached using an open dissection. Then two 2.5 mm trocars are inserted on the line of the anterior border of the sternocleidomastoid muscle 3–4 cm above and below the first incision.[20] Table 3.2 compares these techniques and Figure 3.2 demonstrates the trocars and the positions of the incisions required for these techniques.

All these minimally invasive techniques rely on preoperative localizing studies and may benefit from intraoperative PTH monitoring in certain scenarios as shown by Barczynski et al.[21] The major problem with endoscopic parathyroidectomy is the limited working space so that

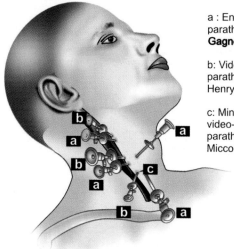

a : Endoscopic parathyroidectomy by **Gagner**

b: Video-assisted parathyroidectomy by Henry

c: Minimally invasive video-assisted parathyroidectomy by Miccoli

Fig. 3.2: Trocar placement in endoscopic approaches to parathyroidectomy.

associated nodular thyroid disease and the presence of a large (> 3 cm) parathyroid adenoma are relative contraindications. It has also been difficult to show a real advantage for endoscopic versus open minimally invasive surgery, largely due to the expense of the endoscopic equipment required. In 2006, Barczynski published a prospective, randomized trial on open versus video-assisted techniques.[22] This showed a preference in the MIVAP group due to an easier recognition of the recurrent laryngeal nerve, less postoperative pain and a better cosmetic result. On the other hand, there was a significantly higher operative cost. Bilateral endoscopic exploration for secondary HPT has been reported with good results.[23,24]

Key Point

- Endoscopic techniques have been shown to be safe but the advantage is minimal.

PARATHYROID CANCER

A literature search of parathyroid cancer reveals more articles on the subject than there are reported cases of the disease. The concern among endocrine surgeons and related specialists is to diagnose the condition accurately and to a lesser extent what operation to perform. Histopathology criteria for the diagnosis of parathyroid cancer were first published in 1973. However, the clinical outcomes of patients diagnosed on these criteria showed that a large number do not clinically progress and the number of reported cases with proven lymph node involvement and metastatic spread outside of the neck is very small, suggesting that these criteria may overdiagnose the condition. DeLellis produced criteria in 2004[25] that defined parathyroid cancer as proven by metastases, adjacent tissue invasion or vascular invasion and anything in between a normal adenoma and carcinoma is an atypical adenoma. There is a wide fluctuation in the reported incidence of parathyroid cancer from 0.5 to 4% of all parathyroid cases.[26] A large series of parathyroid patients looking at the long-term changes in incidence have reported a decline in incidence, since the availability of serum PTH and calcium assays, from 1% pre 1990 to 0.4% now, combined with an increased incidence of parathyroidectomy.[27] This change in incidence could support the concept of a stepwise progression from adenoma to atypical adenoma to carcinoma with fewer cancers appearing as parathyroid disease, which has been detected and treated earlier.[28]

Ippolito et al[27] published follow-up data on the existence of atypical adenomas, which at operation are indistinguishable from carcinoma and reclassified some of the lesions that had been called cancer into atypical adenoma. They showed that 16 of 27 carcinomas were not carcinomas but atypical adenomas, explaining in part the lack of lymph node or distant metastases in parathyroid cancers. In their series, four patients had had a recurrent laryngeal nerve sacrificed, of whom none had perineural invasion on histology and only one had a carcinoma, suggesting a nerve sparing resection, which should be performed in all. None of the atypical adenomas recurred, but four of eleven carcinomas did. Ippolito et al found that en bloc resection did not increase the rate of recurrence or reduce the disease free interval. This finding is contrary to the most previous reports, best summed up by Koea et al,[26] showing en bloc resection had a local recurrence rate of 8% and simple parathyroidectomy had a recurrence rate of 51%.

Key Point

- After local or en bloc resection, once a patient develops a recurrence, cure is not possible.

Recently, the importance of the HRPT 2 gene and parafibromin expression in parathyroid cancer has become better understood and may represent a real advance in the diagnostic markers available to help diagnose the disease more accurately. Loss of parafibromin expression is present in 70% of parathyroid cancers and a tiny percentage of adenomas and atypical adenomas. The HRPT 2 gene encodes parafibromin and thus has other measurable products. Protein gene product (PGP) 9.5 is one such product of the HRPT 2 gene and presence of this protein has 100% specificity for cancer and 78% sensitivity.[29]

Parafibromin and PGP 9.5 may be useful diagnostic markers in those not reaching DeLellis' criteria. Atypical adenoma could be a stage in an adenoma carcinoma sequence. In summary, parathyroid cancer is a rare and probably overdiagnosed and overtreated. Lymph node dissection may not be required as there are no reports of lymph node metastases in parathyroid cancer and efforts to shave tumor off the recurrent laryngeal nerve rather than sacrificing it, is probably oncologically safe. The role of en bloc resection is probably worth adhering to as it may reduce the risk of recurrence in true carcinomas but not at the expense of the recurrent laryngeal nerve. The DeLellis' criteria for classifying parathyroid cancer may avoid over treatment and overdiagnosis, without compromising the risk of recurrence.

CRYOPRESERVATION

Cryopreservation is not a recent advance in itself. Parathyroid tissue was first cryopreserved in the late 1970s for being used in autologous trans-plantation in patients with iatrogenic permanent hypoparathyroidism. However, three papers from 2005,[30] 2008[31] and 2009[32] have added additional useful information on the outcomes of this technique and are worth knowing, as they provide justification for limiting the use and the storage time of cryopreserved tissue, the expense of which is its major drawback.

Cryopreservation has been described in all types of HPT, but the risks of permanent hypoparathyroidism are greatest in multigland disease. Immediate autotransplantation of parathyroid tissue is successful in over 80% of patients. Permanent hypoparathyroidism is rare, affecting approximately 1% of patients that undergo thyroid or parathyroid exploration, but the consequences are difficult to manage (see later); with wide fluctuations in serum calcium producing severe symptoms that are unpredictable. The management of these symptoms, by over-replacing calcium, has metabolic consequences, particularly for renal function and lithiasis (see later).

The drawbacks to cryopreservation are the expense of processing and particularly storing the tissue, as it was not known how long it could be stored for. A paper by Cohen et al showed that at re-implantation 46% of patients have a completely successful transplant and a further 23% have a partially successful transplant, still requiring some calcium supplementation.[30] This result compares favorably with others. A paper from the Mayo Clinic showed that only 23% were off supplementation and only 40% had PTH secretion after re-implanting cryopreserved parathyroid tissue[33] and most recently a French multicenter study showed a complete success of only 10% and failure rate of 80% when cryopreser-vation is performed in small volume centers. Given that only 1.6% of cryopreserved tissue is re-implanted, there are no large centers to compare with.[32] The cause of low success rates with cryopreservation may be the freezing process but it is uncertain how this affects the re-implantation outcome. Cell viability has a key role, as maybe the original parathyroid pathology with hyperplastic tissue is showing greater PTH levels after transplantation than adenomatous tissue.[34] The duration of cryopreservation has not been shown to affect cell viability in in vitro studies,[35,36] but has been shown to affect outcome in clinical studies of re-implanting cryopreserved parathyroid tissue.[30,31] Both papers agree that after a period of two years in storage cryopreserved tissue will not function.

Key Point

- Cryopreserved tissue could be discarded after two years, so that maintaining a tissue bank would become less expensive. Given the limited success of cryopreservation there is also a case for limiting its use to patients with primary multigland disease or not using it at all.

MANAGEMENT OF PERMANENT HYPOCALCEMIA

As outlined earlier, permanent hypocalcemia is rare after thyroid or parathyroid surgery. It is almost impossible to correct serum hypocalcemia in the presence of hypomagnesemia and this should be sought in patients who have hypocalcemia after undergoing neck exploration. Both vitamin D and PTH are integral to calcium homeostasis. Vitamin D increases absorption of calcium from the gut. PTH reduces renal excretion of calcium, mobilizes calcium from the bone and is essential for the hydroxylation of one hydroxycholecalciferol (D3) to 1, 25 di-hyroxycholecalciferal (D4), which is the active component of vitamin D. For this reason giving ergocalciferol or cholecalciferol (D3) to hypoparathyroid, hypocalcemic patients does not work. Instead alpha-calcidol or calcitriol (D4) is required, either 0.5 µg or 1.0 µg per day with two calcium tablets, increasing doses dependent upon serum calcium. The problem is that without PTH there is little selective calcium resorption from the renal nephron so large doses of D4 and calcium to restore serum calcium to the normal range results in hypercalciuria, which causes renal lithiasis and nephrocalcinosis with impairment of renal function. Hence, hypocalcemia resulting from permanent hypoparathyroidism requires specialist management with at least yearly urine calcium measurements and vitamin D dose adjustment accordingly. Thiazide diuretics will also increase resorption of calcium from the nephron and may be used in the treatment of hypoparathyroid hypocalcemia. One should aim to keep the serum calcium at the low range of normal using predominantly vitamin D4 replacement. It is not chronic hypocalcemia that seems to produce symptoms but rapid fluctuations in serum calcium that can precipitate the severe symptoms associated with hypocalcemia.[37] Most recently recombinant PTH administration has been tried in neonatal hypoparathyroidism and psuedo-hypoparathyroidism.[38]

At present, there is an absence of trial results to recommend its use in iatrogenic hypoparathyroidism.

Key Point

- Hypocalcemia resulting from permanent hypoparathyroidism requires specialist management with at least yearly urine calcium measurements and vitamin D dose adjustment accordingly. One should aim to keep the serum calcium at the low range of normal using predominantly vitamin D4 replacement.

REFERENCES

1. Kandil E, Tufaro AP, Carson KA, Lin F, Somervell H, Farrag T, et al. Correlation of plasma 25-hydroxyvitamin D levels with severity of primary HPT and likelihood of parathyroid adenoma localization on sestamibi scan. Arch Otolaryngol Head Neck Surg 2008;134(10):1071-5.
2. BHH Lang, CY Lo. Vitamin D3 deficiency is associated with late onset hypocalcemia after minimally invasive parathyroidectomy in a vitamin D borderline area. Abstract 0360. World J Surg 2009;33(Suppl 1):S141.
3. Skandarajah A, Barlier A, Morlet-Barla N, Sebag F, Enjalbert A, Conte-Devolx B, et al. Should routine analysis of the MEN 1 gene be performed in all patients with primary HPT under 40 years of age? Abstract 0142. World J Surg 2009;33(Suppl 1):S3-259.
4. Cetani F, Pardi E, Borsari S, Viacava P, Dipollina G, Cianferotti L, et al. Genetic analyses of the HRPT2 gene in primary HPT: germline and somatic mutations in familial and sporadic parathyroid tumors. J Clin Endocrinol Metab 2004;89(11):5583-91.
5. Carchman E, Ogilvie J, Holst J, Yim J, Carty S. Appropriate surgical treatment of lithium-associated HPT. World J Surg 2008;32(10):2195-9.
6. Zamani A, Omrani GR, Nasab MM. Lithium's effect on bone mineral density. Bone 2009;44(2):331-4.
7. Hundley JC, Woodrum DT, Saunders BD, Doherty GM, Gauger PG. Revisiting lithium-associated HPT in the era of intraoperative parathyroid hormone monitoring. Surgery 2005;138(6):1027-31; discussion 1031-2.
8. Harrison BJ, Triponez F. Intraoperative adjuncts in surgery for primary HPT. Langenbecks Arch Surg 2009;394(5):799-809.
9. Chan RK, Ibrahim SI, Pil P, Tanasijevic M, Moore FD. Validation of a method to replace frozen section during parathyroid exploration by using the rapid parathyroid hormone assay on parathyroid aspirates. Arch Surg 2005; 140(4):371-3.
10. Lo CY, Chan WF, Leung P, Luk JM. Applicability of tissue aspirate for quick parathyroid hormone assay to confirm parathyroid tissue identity during parathyroidectomy for primary HPT. Arch Surg 2005;140(2):146-9; discussion 150.
11. Perrier ND, Ituarte P, Kikuchi S, Siperstein AE, Duh QY, Clark OH, et al. Intraoperative parathyroid aspiration and parathyroid hormone assay as an alternative to frozen section for tissue identification. World J Surg 2000;24(11):1319-22.

12. Westra WH, Pritchett DD, Udelsman R. Intraoperative confirmation of parathyroid tissue during parathyroid exploration: A retrospective evaluation of the frozen section. Am J Surg Pathol 1998;22(5):538-44.
13. Boggs JE, Irvin GL, Carneiro DM, Molinari AS. The evolution of parathyroidectomy failures. Surgery 1999;126(6):998-1002; discussion 1002-3.
14. Bergenfelz A, Lindblom P, Tibblin S, Westerdahl J. Unilateral versus bilateral neck exploration for primary HPT: a prospective randomized controlled trial. Ann Surg 2002;236(5):543-51.
15. Russell CF, Dolan SJ, Laird JD. Randomized clinical trial comparing scan-directed unilateral versus bilateral cervical exploration for primary HPT due to solitary adenoma. Br J Surg 2006;93(4):418-21.
16. Palazzo FF, Delbridge LW. Minimal-Access/minimally invasive parathyroidectomy for primary HPT. Surg Clin North Am 2004;84(3):717-34.
17. Miccoli P, Berti P, Materazzi G, Donatini G. Minimally invasive video-assisted parathyroidectomy (MIVAP). European Journal of Surgical Oncology 2003;29(2):188-90.
18. Henry JF, Defechereux T, Gramatica L, De Boissezon C. [Endoscopic parathyroidectomy via a lateral neck incision]. Ann Chir 1999;53(4):302-6.
19. Miccoli P, Berti P, Materazzi G, Ambrosini CE, Fregoli L, Donatini G. Endoscopic bilateral neck exploration versus quick intraoperative parathormone assay (qptha) during endoscopic parathyroidectomy: a prospective randomized trial. Surg Endosc 2008;22(2):398-400.
20. Henry JF, Sebag F, Tamagnini P, Forman C, Silaghi H. Endoscopic parathyroid surgery: results of 365 consecutive procedures. World J Surg 2004;28(12):1219-23.
21. Barczynski M, Konturek A, Cichon S, Hubalewska-Dydejczyk A, Golkowski F, Huszno B. Intraoperative parathyroid hormone assay improves outcomes of minimally invasive parathyroidectomy mainly in patients with a presumed solitary parathyroid adenoma and missing concordance of preoperative imaging. Clin Endocrinol (Oxf) 2007;66(6):878-85.
22. Barczyński M, Cichoń S, Konturek A, Cichoń W. Minimally invasive video-assisted parathyroidectomy versus open minimally invasive parathyroidectomy for a solitary parathyroid adenoma: a prospective, randomized, blinded trial. World J Surg 2006;30(5):721-31.
23. Barbaros U, Erbil Y, Yildirim A, Saricam G, Yazici H, Ozarmaðan S. Minimally invasive video-assisted subtotal parathyroidectomy with thymectomy for secondary HPT. Langenbecks Arch Surg 2009;394(3):451-5.
24. Sun Y, Cai H, Bai J, Zhao H, Miao Y. Endoscopic total parathyroidectomy and partial parathyroid tissue autotransplantation for patients with secondary HPT: a new surgical approach. World J Surg 2009;33(8):1674-9.
25. IARC press. DeLellis RA, lloys RV, Heitz PU, Eng C, editors. Lyon: IARC Press; 2004.
26. Koea JB, Shaw JH. Parathyroid cancer: biology and management. Surg Oncol 1999;8(3):155.
27. Ippolito G, Palazzo FF, Sebag F, De Micco C, Henry JF. Intraoperative diagnosis and treatment of parathyroid cancer and atypical parathyroid adenoma. Br J Surg 2007;94(5):566-70.

28. Kirkby-Bott J, Lewis P, Harmer CL, Smellie WJ. One stage treatment of parathyroid cancer. Eur J Surg Oncol 2005;31(1):78-83.

29. Howell VM, Gill A, Clarkson A, Nelson AE, Dunne R, Delbridge LW, et al. Accuracy of combined protein gene product 9.5 and parafibromin markers for immunohistochemical diagnosis of parathyroid carcinoma. J Clin Endocrinol Metab 2009;94(2):434-41.

30. Cohen MS, Dilley WG, Wells SA, Moley JF, Doherty GM, Sicard GA, et al. Long-term functionality of cryopreserved parathyroid autografts: a 13-year prospective analysis. Surgery 2005;138(6):1033-40; discussion 1040-1.

31. Guerrero MA, Evans DB, Lee JE, Bao R, Bereket A, Gantela S, et al. Viability of cryopreserved parathyroid tissue: when is continued storage versus disposal indicated? World J Surg 2008;32(5):836-9.

32. Borot Sophie, Lapierre Valérie, Carnaille Bruno, Goudet Pierre, Penfornis Alfred. Results of cryopreserved parathyroid autografts: a retrospective multicenter study. Surgery 2010.

33. Caccitolo JA, Farley DR, van Heerden JA, Grant CS, Thompson GB, Sterioff S. The current role of parathyroid cryopreservation and autotransplantation in parathyroid surgery: an institutional experience. Surgery 1997;122(6): 1062-7.

34. Goudet P, Cougard P, Zeller V, Brunet-Lecomte P, Viard H. Transplantation of human cryopreserved adenomatous and hyperplastic parathyroid tissue to the hypocalcemic nude mouse. World J Surg 1993;17(5):628-31; discussion 632-3.

35. Herrera MF, Grant CS, van Heerden JA, Jacobsen D, Weaver A, Fitzpatrick LA. The effect of cryopreservation on cell viability and hormone secretion in human parathyroid tissue. Surgery 1992;112(6):1096-101; discussion 1101-2.

36. McHenry CR, Stenger DB, Calandro NK. The effect of cryopreservation on parathyroid cell viability and function. Am J Surg 1997;174(5):481-4.

37. Cooper MS, Gittoes NJL. Diagnosis and management of hypocalcaemia. British Medical Journal 2008;336(7656):1298.

38. Walker Harris V, Jan De Beur S. Postoperative hypoparathyroidism: medical and surgical therapeutic options. Thyroid 2009;19(9):967-73.

SECTION FOUR

UPPER GASTROINTESTINAL (GI)/ HEPATOPANCREATOBILIARY (HPB)

CHAPTER FOUR

Expanding Indications for
Liver Transplantation

Michael A Silva, Peter J Friend

INTRODUCTION AND OVERVIEW

The first liver transplant (LT) was performed by Thomas Starzl in 1963[1] but it was four years before there was a long-term survivor.[2] Liver transplantation in Europe was first performed by Roy Calne in 1968.[3] Throughout the 1970s and 1980s, liver transplantation remained the preserve of a very small group of pioneers who struggled with surgical and immunological problems leading to poor long-term results.[4]

The rapid expansion of liver transplantation, which took place during the 1980s was due to the advent of newer immunosuppression, particularly cyclosporine, which enabled lower levels of rejection to be achieved while reducing the doses of steroids needed.[5] Later, in the 1990s, further new drugs contributed to improving results, particularly tacrolimus[6] and mycophenolate.[7] The efficacy of organ preservation was substantially improved with the introduction of University of Wisconsin solution at around the same time.[8] These benefits, combined with incremental improvements in surgical, anesthetic and postoperative care resulted in a massive improvement in the outcome of liver transplantation between 1980 and 2000.

Liver transplantation was formally acknowledged as an effective therapy for endstage liver disease at an NIH consensus meeting in June 1983[9,10] and was rapidly adopted by an increasing number of transplant units around the world. In recent years, 1-year and 5-year survival figures of 90% and 75% have been achieved. This success has inspired management guidelines for patients with liver disease that recommend that every patient with endstage liver disease be referred for liver transplant assessment.[11] While the number of patients awaiting liver transplantation has therefore steadily increased, there has been no corresponding increase in the number of organs available for transplantation. Since 2000, the number of livers transplanted internationally has stabilized for this reason (European Liver Transplant Association (ELTA) website). In the USA, there are currently approximately 16,000 patients on the liver transplant waiting list and just over 6,300 liver transplants were performed in 2008 as per UNOS (United Network for Organ Sharing, September, 2009).

In the UK, there is currently a mortality of about 6% of patients on the waiting list while a further 6% of patients are removed from the waiting list having become too sick to withstand the process of a transplant (National Health Service Blood and Transplant (NHSBT) data). UK data from March 2009 shows 667 patients transplanted in the previous year and 338 patients on the active transplant waiting list. A pattern of increasing waiting list size, static transplant rates and increasing waiting list mortality is common not only in the UK and USA, but also in the most countries across the world.

For this reason, a major focus of attention over the last 10 years has been that of organ allocation—how to achieve the most benefit from the limited number of donor organs that are available while still retaining a system based on fairness. Such allocation systems are complex and based on a variety of parameters, including waiting time, urgency (life expectancy without transplant) and likely benefit (life expectancy after transplantation). As might be expected, a range of allocation systems has evolved in different countries.

Surgical developments continue to play an important part in the evolution of liver transplantation, particularly in the quest for novel sources of donor organs. Developments in liver resection surgery led directly to the ability to split one healthy donor liver into two components, both suitable for transplantation into separate recipients. This was first applied successfully in the case of one small (pediatric) recipient of the left lobe or (more commonly) left lateral segment and one large (adult) recipient of the right lobe. As waiting list mortality increasingly affects the adult waiting list, the current drive is to apply this to two adult recipients.

The success of surgical techniques for liver reduction and liver splitting led to the development of living donor liver transplantation. This was carried out initially in those countries in which cadaveric donation is not widely available for legal or cultural reasons but where liver disease is prevalent and high-level skills in liver resection are available. It has become more widely practiced in Western countries but concerns about donor safety have resulted in some reduction in support for this procedure.

The increasing demand for donor organs over the last two decades has coincided with important changes in the nature of the donor population in most countries. An increasing proportion of cadaveric donors are patients who have suffered a cerebrovascular catastrophe: This is matched by a decreasing proportion of donors who have been declared brain dead following cerebral trauma (largely due to a welcome reduction in road deaths in most developed countries). Donors are, therefore, on average older and have more comorbid disease. A substantial proportion of potential liver donors has significant steatosis, which is very common in patients on intensive care units. Moderate or severe steatosis of the donor liver is now well-recognized to have a detrimental effect on the outcome following liver transplantation. It is a major challenge of the current era to develop means to transplant successfully these and other 'marginal' donor organs.

Another important potential source of additional donor organs is the use of 'non-heartbeating' donors. Conventionally, organ donors for liver transplantation are those declared brain-dead following rigorous neurological testing. Such 'heartbeating' donors have intact circulation while lung function is maintained by mechanical ventilation and it is, therefore, possible to remove the donor organs with minimal warm ischemia (the period between circulatory arrest and *in situ* cooling of the organs). In donors, whom death is declared following cardiac arrest, there is an inevitable period between circulatory arrest and organ cooling. This period of warm ischemia compounds the subsequent period of preservation (cold ischemia) and leads to more substantial reperfusion damage at the time of implantation. Partly as a result of changes in the management of patients with intracranial catastrophes and partly as a result of the drive to increase the referral of all possible organ donors, the number of non-heartbeating donors is increasing. Much research effort is currently being directed to novel methods by which livers from such donors can be safely and effectively transplanted.

DEMAND MANAGEMENT AND ORGAN ALLOCATION

In order to reconcile the availability of donor organs with the demand, it is necessary to regulate which patients are placed on the waiting list and the allocation of the donor organs to patients on the list. Different countries implement this in different ways, but with the same overall intention that there should be a consistent approach to offering liver transplantation and that organ allocation should be equitable.

With respect to placing patients on the waiting list, in the USA, minimal listing criteria was agreed at a consensus conference at the National Institute of Health organized by the American Society of Transplant Physicians (AST) and the American Association for the Study of Liver Disease (AASLD) in 1996[12] (Table 4.1). These criteria define the minimum severity of liver disease for which liver transplantation can be offered (preventing a patient from being listed at too early a stage in the disease). In the UK, there is an agreement that no patient should be listed if the prognosis following liver transplantation is worse than a 50% survival at five years (preventing a patient from being listed with liver disease that is too advanced or for a condition that does not respond well to transplantation).

TABLE 4.1

Minimal listing criteria for liver transplantation (non-disease specific)

Immediate need for liver transplantation

- Estimated 1 year survival without transplantation of less than 90%.
- Childs-Pugh score of 7 or greater (Childs class B or C).
- History of bleeding from portal hypertension or spontaneous bacterial peritonitis (irrespective of Childs score).

Regarding allocation, in the USA, this is based on the model for end-stage liver disease (MELD), in order to give priority to the sickest patients.[13] Based on three biochemical variables,[1] serum bilirubin,[2] serum creatinine[3] and coagulation (international normalized ratio), this has been shown in retrospective and prospective studies to be highly predictive of 3-month mortality in patients with chronic liver disease (Table 4.2). Similarly, for patients of less than 12 years of age, the PELD model has been shown retrospectively to be predictive of waiting list mortality; this incorporates height, weight and serum albumin as predictive parameters.

Clearly the MELD system does not cater for patients in whom urgency is due to malignancy rather than parenchymal liver function. Once acceptable listing criteria for transplantation of patients with hepatocellular carcinoma were agreed (see below), these patients were then awarded an (arbitrary) MELD score to reflect their state of clinical urgency.

TABLE 4.2

Model for end-stage liver disease (MELD) scoring system

- Serum creatinine (Log$_e$ value) 0.957
  - The maximum serum creatinine considered within the MELD score equation is 4.0 mg/dL (i.e. for candidates with a serum creatinine >4.0 mg/dL, the serum creatinine level is set to 4.0 mg/dL).
  - For candidates on dialysis, defined as having two or more dialysis treatments within the prior week or candidates who have received 24 hours of continuous veno-venous hemodialysis (CVVHD) within the prior week, the serum creatinine level is automatically be set to 4.0 mg/dL.
- Serum bilirubin (Log$_e$ value) 0.378
- International normalized ratio (INR) (Log$_e$ value) 1.120
- Using these prognostic factors and regression coefficients, the UNetSM computerized system assigns a MELD score for each candidate based on the following calculation: MELD score = 0.957 x Log$_e$ (creatinine mg/dL) + 0. 378 x Log$_e$ (bilirubin mg/dL) + 1.120 x Log$_e$ (INR) + 0.643. Laboratory values <1.0 are set to 1.0 for the purposes of the MELD score calculation.
- The MELD score for each liver transplant candidate derived from this calculation is rounded to the tenth decimal place and then multiplied by 10.
- The MELD score is limited to a total of 40 points maximum.

The initial algorithm, introduced in 2002 was modified such that patients with a T2 lesion are currently listed with a MELD score of 22.[14]

In the UK, there are two categories of patient on the waiting list. 'Super-urgent' patients are those who have a high probability of death if not transplanted within three days – due to fulminant liver failure, primary non-function of a transplanted liver or hepatic arterial thrombosis within three weeks following a liver transplant. Such patients have absolute priority for any donor liver of compatible blood type; if there is more than one such patient for a given liver, then priority is based on the time of listing. All other donor livers are allocated to the unit rather than the patient (based on the retrieval zone) and allocation is based on local criteria. However, with the increasing discrepancy between supply and demand and the resulting increasing mortality on the waiting list, there is great pressure to introduce national allocation for all organs in order to ensure equity of access to every patient, irrespective of the transplant unit at which the patient is registered.

INDICATIONS FOR LIVER TRANSPLANTATION

Liver transplantation may be required for four main reasons: chronic liver failure, fulminant liver failure, inherited metabolic liver disease and liver tumors.

With increasing experience, the list of contraindications for transplantation has been refined and shortened. Many contraindications that were once considered absolute are now seen as relative: these include portal vein thrombosis, chronic renal failure, hepatopulmonary syndrome, porto pulmonary hypertension and HIV seropositivity. Advanced age is no longer considered an absolute contraindication – physiological rather than chronological, age dictates the individual's suitability. Severe obesity once considered an absolute is now a relative contraindication. Conditions that remain absolute contraindications include HIV AIDS, extra-hepatic malignancy (exceptions to this rule include metastatic neuroendocrine malignancies); active untreated sepsis; advanced cardiopulmonary disease; active alcohol or substance abuse.[9]

In recent years there has been continued debate as to the best management of patients with alcoholic liver disease, chronic viral hepatitis B and C, hepatic malignancy and patients with HIV.

Alcoholic Liver Disease

Liver transplantation for patients with alcoholic liver disease raises issues and controversies not seen in patients with other indications. This is partly based on the perception that alcoholic liver disease is self induced (despite the fact that clear genetic and environmental influences exist), but mainly because the recipient may return to a pattern of drinking that will damage the graft. At the time of transplantation, most if not all transplant candidates have stopped drinking.[15] Appropriate screening has been shown to detect all but the most determined of alcoholics. The length of abstinence before transplantation does not reliably predict abstinence afterwards; there is, therefore, little justification for a fixed arbitrary period of abstinence before transplantation.[16] However, a period of abstinence may identify patients in whom recovery of liver function may occur and so obviate the need for transplantation. It may also allow time to explore psychological and social issues and to put in place strategies to prevent a return to previous patterns of misuse.

Serious concerns, however, remain about the place of transplantation for patients with alcoholic hepatitis (rather than cirrhosis); this is partly because the survival without transplantation is so short that a full assessment often not possible. There are also anxieties about those patients who have consistently failed to change their drinking behavior or to engage with addiction services.[15]

After transplantation 8 to 22% of patients relapse (consumption of any amount of alcohol) within six months and 10 to 30% relapse overall.[17] This compares with conventional treatment for alcohol dependence in which a 60 to 80% relapse rate at two years is expected. It is, therefore, more appropriate to ask not whether patients with alcoholic liver disease should receive transplants but whether enough is being done to provide support after a successful operation.[15]

Despite concerns that patients with alcoholic liver disease may resume drinking after transplantation, the graft survival rate in patients with alcoholic liver disease is comparable to that of patients with non-alcoholic liver disease (UNOS 2002). In fact, the 1- and 3-year graft-survival rates in such patients are above the average graft-survival rates for all diagnoses.[15]

Chronic Viral Hepatitis

The pandemic of chronic viral hepatitis accounts for more patients awaiting liver transplantation than any other single indication. The worldwide prevalence of hepatitis C is estimated to be about 3% and approximately 1.8% of the population of the US is infected. Mortality from hepatitis C is expected to increase by 3 to 5-fold over the next two decades.[18]

Hepatitis C and Liver Transplantation

When antiviral therapy fails in hepatitis C virus infection, or if diagnosis of the disease is delayed until the appearance of end-stage liver disease with portal hypertension, the only option for the individual is liver replacement.[19] Unfortunately, liver transplantation is not a cure for hepatitis C because viral recurrence is inevitable leading to damage of the new liver. Recurrent hepatitis C infection is among the most frequent causes of graft loss and the need for retransplantation. Viral control before and after transplantation in order to mitigate the progress of recurrent disease represents one of the major challenges in managing this group of patients.

In patients with active hepatitis C and viral replication before transplantation, recurrent viremia after transplantation is universal. Attempts to prevent re-infection with immunoglobulin or other agents have not been successful. Re-infection occurs during reperfusion of the liver allograft and viral titers reach pre-transplant values by about 72 hours. At steady state, the hepatitis C viral load is, in general, ten times higher after transplantation than before. Histological evidence of recurrence with allograft hepatitis owing to hepatitis C occurs in up to 90% of individuals by the fifth year after transplantation.[19]

Most studies have shown that the severity of recurrent hepatitis C is similar irrespective of whether cyclosporine- or tacrolimus-based immunosuppression is used. It appears to be the overall intensity of immunosuppression that affects outcomes; more intense treatment leads to worse outcomes. Usual practice is therefore to select adequate immunosuppression to minimize the incidence of rejection, followed by a very gradual taper and to avoid intense treatment for rejection with bolus doses of steroids or antibodies.[19]

The issue of retransplantation for recurrent hepatitis C is controversial and the strategies of different units vary widely; some centers no longer perform this because of poor outcomes. Individuals undergoing retransplantation for hepatitis C have worse outcomes than those undergoing primary transplantations; however, the outcomes are not clearly worse than those after retransplantation for other causes.

Hepatitis B and Liver Transplantation

Liver transplantation is an excellent mode of treatment for hepatitis B virus infected patients who have acute or chronic liver failure and/or primary liver cancer. Advances in antiviral prophylaxis with lamivudine and adefovir now prevent clinically significant graft re-infection for the majority of patients. Graft and patient survival have improved greatly during the past decade and results of transplantation for hepatitis B virus are now superior to those achieved for most other indications.[20]

Transplants that do become re-infected with hepatitis B also respond well to combination nucleoside analog therapy, which can achieve sustained suppression of viral replication. Hepatitis B antigen and hepatitis B surface antigen clearance are also observed.[20]

Hepatic Malignancy

Although primary liver cancer was initially an indication for liver transplantation, it soon became clear that the recurrence rate was very high. As the shortage of donor organs became severe during the 1990s, it was agreed that a relatively non-selective approach to the transplantation of patients with primary liver tumors could no longer be justified in terms of best utilization of scarce organs.

Hepatocellular Cancer (HCC)

Application of more stringent criteria regarding tumor size and number produced superior results[21] and further investigation produced criteria (a single lesion up to 5 cm or up to 3 smaller lesions with none greater than 3 cm) that achieved acceptable rates of recurrence: these Milan criteria[22] have been widely implemented.

Candidates with HCC are often treated with loco-regional therapy while undergoing evaluation or waiting for transplantation in order to limit the growth of disease. Commonly used treatments include radiofrequency ablation (RFA) and transarterial chemoembolization (TACE). A number of single-center reports have indicated that these techniques may be beneficial in preventing tumor progression beyond the Milan criteria. Although this does have the advantage that the patient remains within approved criteria and therefore retains priority,[14,23,24] there are no randomized controlled prospective data to show that these techniques are of definitive value. Nonetheless, almost all transplant centers perform these ablative procedures and in increasing numbers.

A number of centers have carried out transplantation in patients beyond the Milan criteria (although in the USA these patients often do not receive MELD priority scores). Several single-center reports have shown that the Milan criteria can be incrementally expanded without paying a penalty with regard to recurrence.[14] Of the various criteria that have been studied, the most widely accepted are the University of California San Francisco (UCSF) criteria with a limit based on: 1 nodule ≤ 6.5 cm or 2–3 nodules ≤ 4.5 cm and total tumor diameter ≤ 8 cm. These have been independently validated.[14,25,26] It is clear that the tumor mass is a continuous variable in relation to risk of recurrence and the further the criteria are expanded beyond Milan, the higher the price that is paid in terms of patient survival and recurrence.[27,28]

Many transplant centers now believe the Milan criteria to be excessively conservative and in the USA, two UNOS regions have agreed MELD priority scores for lesions that meet specific criteria beyond those of Milan (Fig. 4.1); preliminary results are encouraging.[14]

One of the intrinsic problems of basing patient eligibility on the Milan criteria is that these are based on preoperative radiological staging and

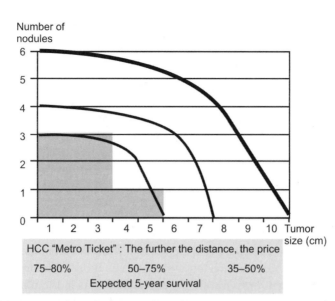

Fig. 4.1: Beyond the Milan Criteria. The HCC *"Metro Ticket"* the University of California, San Francisco (UCSF). This graph depicts five-year survival figures in relation to the Milan criteria and beyond.[31] HCCs that are within the Milan criteria have an overall 5-year survival in the region of 75 to 80% post-transplantation. Those within the UCSF criteria have an overall 5-year survival of approximately 50 to 75%. When the criteria are expanded even beyond this the price paid is a lower long-term survival.

cannot take account of the nature of tumor biology, vascular or lymphatic invasion etc. Other tumor characteristics are known to predict a high-risk for tumor recurrence; these include poorly differentiated grade and high alpha-fetoprotein levels.[29] In addition, response to down-staging may serve as a prognostic marker and may help select a subgroup with more favorable biology for liver transplantation.[30]

Cholangiocarcinoma (CCA)

In the 1980s and early 1990s, there was considerable enthusiasm for transplantation for primary liver cancers, including cholangiocarcinoma. The University of Pittsburgh was the first to report a disappointing 2-year survival of 30% and a prohibitive disease recurrence rate of 60%.[32] Others also reported high patient mortality owing to disease recurrence leading to a consensus among most units that transplantation is not appropriate treatment for cholangiocarcinoma.[33,34]

In leading centers worldwide, the standard surgical strategy for hilar cholangiocarcinoma is therefore extensive liver resection. However, the reported 5-year survival rates of 20 to 30% are far from encouraging.[35] Clearly an effective therapy for this condition is much needed and a strategy based on transplantation has many attractions. Since 1993, at the Mayo Clinic, a selected group of patients with unresectable hilar CCA was subjected to a novel protocol, which combined radiotherapy, chemosensitization and liver transplantation. A combination of external beam radiotherapy and intravenous fluorouracil was supplemented with iridium wire brachytherapy prior to a staging operation.

Only patients with operatively confirmed stage I or II disease underwent liver transplantation.[36] Very impressive results were reported from this highly selected group of patients, with one, three and 5-year patient survival rates of 92%, 82% and 82% respectively. This protocol for the treatment of non-resectable hilar CCA has not yet been replicated elsewhere or reached broader application.

Liver Transplantation in Patients with HIV

Because these diseases share risk factors and route of transmission, many patients with HIV are co-infected with hepatitis B or C. The introduction of highly active antiretroviral therapy (HAART) has led to a spectacular improvement in the survival of patients infected with HIV. For this reason, chronic viral hepatitis has become an important cause of death in patients with HIV in recent years.

Although data on the outcome of liver transplantation in HIV-infected recipients with liver disease is limited, the overall results appear comparable to those in non-HIV-infected recipients. Therefore, liver transplant centers around the world are increasingly accepting HIV-infected individuals as suitable candidates for liver transplantation. In addition to the traditional criteria used for transplant eligibility, HIV patients have stricter inclusion criteria for consideration and enrollment (Table 4.3). Post-transplantation control of HIV replication is achieved by continuing HAART. Hepatitis B virus recurrence is effectively prevented by hepatitis B immunoglobulin and antiviral therapy. In the absence of effective antiviral therapy, however, re-infection of the allograft with hepatitis C virus remains an important problem, and progression to allograft cirrhosis may even be more rapid than in HIV-negative patients. Interactions between the HAART and immunosuppressive drugs are difficult to predict and require close monitoring of drug levels. The added

TABLE 4.3

Criteria used for transplant eligibility in HIV patients

Inclusion criteria	Exclusion criteria
• Life expectancy greater than 5 years	• Presence of any cancer diagnosis
• CD4 cell count greater than 200 for over 6 months pre-transplant	• Any untreated chronic illness (including tuberculosis)
• Adherence to stable HAART regimen	• Greater than three classes of viral resistance
• Absence of any AIDS defining illness	
• Plasma viral load less than 50 copies/ml	• Persistent HIV viremia
	• Any non-compliance with HAART

complexity of these various factors necessitates close cooperation between transplant surgeons, hepatologists, HIV-clinicians and pharmacologists.[37,38]

SURGICAL DEVELOPMENTS TO INCREASE DONOR NUMBERS

Split Liver Grafts

A single cadaveric donor liver can be split in order to be used in more than one recipient. Liver splitting for transplantation is based on the following: (i) the lobar anatomic structure of the liver allows for separation of functionally independent units, (ii) the high functional reserve of the healthy liver ensures that 30 to 40% of standard organ mass is sufficient to support life, (iii) the liver's strong regenerative capacity and (iv) the increased experience of liver surgeons in the procedure. The emphasis is therefore on the usage of optimum quality donor livers from for example, young donors with a short stay on intensive treatment unit (ITU) after brain death who have minimal steatosis and none of the other factors that would define the graft as marginal (see below).

Despite the obvious potential for technical problems, particularly related to the biliary and vascular anatomy, in the most experienced units, the outcomes have been shown to be equivalent to those of whole grafts.[39;40] This may be partly related to the selection of the best donor livers for this procedure.

The first application of split liver transplantation was to enable one liver to be transplanted into an adult and a child. This offers a significant advantage to pediatric recipients in terms of life years gained compared with remaining on the waiting list.[41] Splitting for two adults requires high technical skills and knowledge of the anatomic variations and is usually performed in centers with the most experience. With rigid selection criteria, it is feasible to achieve this without an increase in technical complications, delay in allograft function or compromise in patient and graft survival.[42,43]

In 1989, Bismuth was the first to perform liver transplantation to two adult patients from one donor liver to treat two simultaneous cases of fulminant hepatitis.[44] Since then various techniques have been described. The liver can be divided *ex situ* following retrieval from the donor or *in situ* while still perfused in the donor. The advantage of *in situ* split is mainly that the ischemia time is reduced and better hemostasis can be achieved on the cut surface of the liver.

Splitting the liver along the line of Cantilie results in a full right lobe (segments V to VIII) and a full left lobe (segment I to IV), thereby creating two medium-sized grafts for implantation. However, due to the large resection plane in the middle of the liver, special anatomical issues arise in relation to (i) the middle hepatic vein and (ii) the biliary anatomy.

i. If the middle hepatic vein stays with the left lobe, good venous drainage is achieved of segments II to IV via the middle and left hepatic vein draining into the inferior vena cava (IVC). However, segments V and VIII of the right lobe graft are likely to be congested since these are drained predominantly by the middle hepatic vein. Of the several techniques described to overcome this problem the commonest is to anastomose the segment V and VIII veins at the resection plane to a length of donor iliac vein, which acts as a conduit to the recipient IVC. Another problem occurs with venous drainage of the caudate lobe (segment I) as part of a left lobe graft if the IVC remains with the right lobe graft as this segment normally drains directly into the IVC.

ii. Biliary complications, bile leaks and biliary strictures, occur in about 30% of recipients. This is much more frequent than in cadaveric whole liver transplantation. Where it can be achieved, duct-to-duct biliary reconstruction has been shown to be preferable to hepatico-jejunostomy.

Liver Volume in Split Liver Transplantation

The liver represents approximately 5% of body weight in infancy, thereafter decreasing to approximately 2.5% in adults. However, a functional liver mass of 0.8% of body weight is what is required for survival.

The process of splitting a liver does have a detrimental effect on liver function (due to ischemia, cut surface complications and biliary complications) and it is recommended that a lower limit of liver volume of approximately 1% of body weight is realistic for successful transplantation.[45,46] When a graft is less than 0.8% of body weight, small-for-size syndrome is likely to occur. This is due to perfusion of a small liver by a higher than physiological portal venous flow, which results in congestion of the graft with hepatocellular injury, cholestasis, ascites and finally graft failure. There is also an increased incidence of surgical complications, such as intra-abdominal hemorrhage and intestinal perforations. In this setting, regeneration of the liver graft does not occur.

Live Donor Liver Transplantation

A patient is now more likely to die on the waiting list for transplantation than postoperatively. Lengthening waiting lists and increasing waiting list mortality have led patients and transplant surgeons to search further for alternatives to traditional cadaveric organ donors. This pressure has always been greater in those parts of the world where cadaveric organ donation is not widely practiced; this has led to the development of live donor liver transplantation (LDLT) as a viable alternative to cadaveric donor liver transplantation.[47]

In many parts of Asia, particularly Hong Kong, Taiwan, Korea and Japan, the availability of cadaveric donors has always been very low for a number of reasons. Cultural beliefs in many Asian countries have not adapted to the concept of brain-death in the way that Western cultures have done.[48] In Japan until 1997, it was illegal to remove organs from a heart-beating donor. However, the change in the law has had relatively little impact on the availability of cadaveric donors, illustrating that cultural change can be harder to achieve than legal change. There has been little political support for cadaveric transplantation in the form of economic and infrastructure resources. Similarly, in China guidelines for establishing the diagnosis of brain death were drawn up in 2003 but a regulated national network for the transplantation of cadaveric organs is not yet fully established. In India, the Transplantation of Human Organs Bill became law in 1995, legalizing cadaveric organ donation from brain dead donors, but, nonetheless 90% of liver transplants in India still occur using live donor livers.

Live donor liver transplantation developed where the need was strongest and where there were the technical skills and health care resources appropriate to a very demanding surgical procedure. Enormous levels of experience have been accrued in centers first in Japan[49] and later Hong Kong[50] and South Korea.[51] Outside South East Asia, a number of units built up considerable experience in the USA, Europe and elsewhere. Concerns about donor safety were expressed at an early stage and indeed reports of donor mortality did start to appear, albeit at low levels—the currently quoted risk of death is 0.2% to 0.5% (UNOS data). Additionally, morbidity in the donor following surgery is currently reported at 10% to 30%. A series of complications and at least two well-publicized donor deaths in America led to a reassessment of health policy and a very public debate on the subject.[47] This was followed by a reduction in the number of such procedures carried out in the USA.

Early live donor resections were of the left lobe for transplantation into a child or small adult—the risks to the donor of this procedure were felt to be significantly less than on a full right liver lobe because of the larger residual liver mass remaining in the donor. Whereas the left lobe is adequate for a small adult, in order to be able to transplant larger adults successfully using current techniques, a large graft is needed. The safety and the feasibility of right lobe resections from living donors was established by Fan et al.[46]

Certain states in the USA have prohibited live liver donation for recipients with MELD scores of greater than 25. This recommendation was based on: (i) speculation that the outcome of transplantation would be poorer if the recipient received a partial graft and (ii) reservations about the ethics of live donation in circumstances when the mortality of the recipient is intrinsically higher. Nonetheless, excellent outcomes have been reported in recipients with high MELD scores.[52] Complications in the recipient, additional to those seen with whole graft liver transplantation following live donor liver transplantation, are similar to those seen with split liver transplantation.

Marginal and Non-Heartbeating Donor Organs

In an attempt to respond to the growing need for donor grafts, the use of *marginal grafts* has become commonplace. A marginal graft can be defined as an organ with an increased risk for poor function or failure that may subject the recipient to greater risks of morbidity or mortality. There is no consensus however about the specific factors that define a graft as a marginal or about which factors should exclude a particular donor organ. The decision to transplant an organ therefore depends on the judgment of the transplant surgeon and consideration of the details of the specific recipient, as well as donor.[53,54]

Broadly there are two categories of marginal grafts. Firstly, there are grafts which carry a high risk of technical complications and impaired function: examples of these are steatotic livers, organs from non-heart-beating donors (NHBD), elderly donors, split liver grafts, organs from donors with high inotrope requirement or those with long preservation times. The second category is of organs that carry an increased risk of transmission of infection or malignancy to the recipient (Table 4.4). It is the first category that will be discussed below.

The key to the use of marginal donor grafts is risk analysis; what is the prognosis of the particular donor organ transplanted into a particular recipient and what is the risk to the recipient if the transplant does not go ahead? This leads to complex decision-making: it is widely felt, for example that a marginal donor organ should be transplanted into a low-risk recipient because a high-risk recipient (with very advanced liver

TABLE 4.4

Types of marginal grafts

Risk of impaired graft function	Risk of disease transmission
Steatotic livers	Donors with positive serology
Donor obesity	Active bacterial infections
Elderly donors	Unexplained cause of death
Non-heartbeating donor	Donors with malignancy
Grafts from split livers	High-risk lifestyle
Inotropic support	
High serum sodium	
Cardiac arrest	
Long ischemia	
Long ITU stay	

failure) would not survive the postoperative period with anything other than an ideal liver. However, the low-risk recipient is best placed to wait for an ideal liver. Such considerations have increased the complexity of the management of liver transplant waiting lists and local organ allocation decisions and have organizational and ethical dimensions.

While the increased use of marginal grafts has been driven primarily by the critical shortage of donor organs for transplantation, in fact recent results show that marginal grafts can be used with favorable outcomes.[53,54]

Non-Heartbeating Donors (NHBD)

The last decade has seen a considerable renewal of interest in non-heart-beating donors (NHBD) (otherwise referred to as donation after cardiac death), as a means to increase the pool of available organs. This followed the excellent results of kidney transplantation from NHBD and a rapid expansion of NHBD kidney programs in many countries.

NHBDs are described in two broad categories subdivided into four categories according to the 'Maastricht classification' (Table 4.5).[55] 'Uncontrolled' donors are those in whom unpredicted cardiac arrest has occurred either outside the hospital (Maastricht I) or in the hospital (Maastricht II). 'Controlled' donors are those in which cardiac arrest is predicted, following withdrawal of vital support (ventilator or inotropic) on the grounds of futility (Maastricht III). In such cases, the timing is partly predictable based on the time of withdrawal of support and the retrieval team can be presented and prepared. The critical warm ischemia time is, therefore, substantially shorter in such cases. It is this category of NHBD that has been almost exclusively used in liver transplantation although a few units have run programs with uncontrolled NHBD.[56]

The results of liver transplantation from NHBD are inferior to those of heart-beating donor organs with a significantly higher risk of graft failure (relative risk 1.85[57]). A number of risk factors have been identified in multivariate analysis, these include: warm ischemia time greater than 15 minutes; cold preservation time greater than 10 hours; donor age greater than 45 years.[58] The incidence of late-onset, non-anastomotic biliary strictures has proved a major cause for concern, occurring in up to one third of patients. Despite this, excellent results can be obtained with up to 87% graft survival at 12 months,[59] but this required a highly selective

TABLE 4.5

Maastricht classification of NHBD[60]

I	Brought in dead	uncontrolled
II	Unsuccessful resuscitation	
III	Awaiting cardiac arrest	controlled
IV	Cardiac arrest after brain-stem death	

approach to donor selection: 45% of retrieved organs were discarded. There is a great deal to be gained by innovative strategies that enable a wider spectrum of such donor organs be transplanted successfully. Results from uncontrolled NHBD are less good with graft survival at 2 years of 55%.[56]

THE FUTURE

The outcome following liver transplantation has improved progressively throughout the last decade despite the use of less ideal donor organs. The major challenges in the decade ahead will be (i) the donor shortage and (ii) the increasing incidence of hepatitis C-related liver failure.

Increased use of marginal donor organs will make significant inroads to the donor organ shortage, particularly if this includes the widespread use of NHBD organs and of livers with steatosis. Novel approaches to graft assessment, preservation and resuscitation might render a wide range of organs usable that are currently discarded or not considered for transplantation. The evolution of techniques of 'normothermic recirculation[61] and normothermic preservation[62] might not only render damaged organs transplantable but could also provide viability assessment that reduces the risk of primary graft non-function.

The refinement and widespread adoption of techniques for the reliable splitting of donor livers, providing for two adult recipients, will also substantially increase the availability of liver transplantation for increasing numbers of patients.

Molecular and genetic techniques to prevent the re-infection of transplanted livers with hepatitis C are likely to evolve; this would improve the survival and reduce the need for retransplantation of this expanding group of patients.

Liver transplantation benefits many thousands of patients each year around the world; these current challenges are a reflection of its therapeutic success.

REFERENCES

1. Starzl TE, Marchioro TL, Faris TD. Liver transplantation. Ann Intern Med 1966;64(2):473-7.
2. Starzl TE, Groth CG, Brettschneider L, Penn I, Fulginiti VA, Moon JB, et al. Orthotopic homotransplantation of the human liver. Ann Surg 1968; 168(3):392-415.
3. Calne RY. Liver transplantation. Transplant Rev 1969;2:69-89.
4. Williams R, Neuberger J, Calne RY. Current status of liver transplantation. Indian J Gastroenterol 1985;4(4):265-9.
5. White DJ, Calne RY. The use of Cyclosporin A immunosuppression in organ grafting. Immunol Rev 1982;65:115-31.

6. Neuhaus P, Langrehr JM, Williams R, Calne RY, Pichlmayr R, McMaster P. Tacrolimus-based immunosuppression after liver transplantation: a randomised study comparing dual versus triple low-dose oral regimens. Transpl Int 1997;10(4):253-61.

7. McDiarmid SV. Mycophenolate mofetil in liver transplantation. Clin Transplant 1996;10(1 Pt 2):140-5.

8. Jamieson NV, Sundberg R, Lindell S, Claesson K, Moen J, Vreugdenhil PK, et al. The 24- to 48-hour preservation of canine liver by simple cold storage using UW lactobionate solution. Transplant Proc 1989;21(1 Pt 2):1292-3.

9. Maddrey WC, Schieff EW, Sorrel MF, (Eds). Transplantation of the Liver. In Keeffe EB, (Ed). Selection of patients for Liver Transplant. Philadelphia, USA, Lippincott Williams and Wilkins 2001;35-46.

10. McMaster P, Jurewicz WA, Gunson BK, Clements D, Kirby RM, Angrisani L. The current state of liver and pancreas transplantation. Scand J Gastroenterol Suppl 1985;117:69-79.

11. Perera MT, Mirza DF, Elias E. Liver transplantation: Issues for the next 20 years. J Gastroenterol Hepatol 2009;24(Suppl 3):S124-31.

12. Lucey MR, Brown KA, Everson GT, Fung JJ, Gish R, Keeffe EB, et al. Minimal criteria for placement of adults on the liver transplant waiting list: a report of a national conference organized by the American Society of Transplant Physicians and the American Association for the Study of Liver Diseases. Liver Transpl Surg 1997;3(6):628-37.

13. Kanwal F, Dulai GS, Spiegel BM, Yee HF, Gralnek IM. A comparison of liver transplantation outcomes in the pre- vs. post-MELD eras. Aliment Pharmacol Ther 2005;21(2):169-77.

14. Washburn K. Model for End Stage Liver Disease and hepatocellular carcinoma: a moving target. Transplant Rev (Orlando) 2010;24(1):11-7.

15. Webb K, Neuberger J. Transplantation for alcoholic liver disease. BMJ 2004; 329(7457):63-4.

16. Neuberger J, Schulz KH, Day C, Fleig W, Berlakovich GA, Berenguer M, et al. Transplantation for alcoholic liver disease. J Hepatol 2002;36(1):130-7.

17. Perney P, Bismuth M, Sigaud H, Picot MC, Jacquet E, Puche P, et al. Are preoperative patterns of alcohol consumption predictive of relapse after liver transplantation for alcoholic liver disease? Transpl Int 2005;18(11):1292-7.

18. Yen T, Keeffe EB, Ahmed A. The epidemiology of hepatitis C virus infection. J Clin Gastroenterol 2003;36(1):47-53.

19. Brown RS. Hepatitis C and liver transplantation. Nature 2005;436(7053): 973-8.

20. Mutimer D. Review article: hepatitis B and liver transplantation. Aliment Pharmacol Ther 2006;23(8):1031-41.

21. Bismuth H, Chiche L, Adam R, Castaing D, Diamond T, Dennison A. Liver resection versus transplantation for hepatocellular carcinoma in cirrhotic patients. Ann Surg 1993;218(2):145-51.

22. Mazzaferro V, Regalia E, Doci R, Andreola S, Pulvirenti A, Bozzetti F, et al. Liver transplantation for the treatment of small hepatocellular carcinomas in patients with cirrhosis. N Engl J Med 1996;334(11):693-9.

23. Mazzaferro V, Battiston C, Perrone S, Pulvirenti A, Regalia E, Romito R, et al. Radiofrequency ablation of small hepatocellular carcinoma in cirrhotic

patients awaiting liver transplantation: a prospective study. Ann Surg 2004; 240(5):900-9.

24. Millonig G, Graziadei IW, Freund MC, Jaschke W, Stadlmann S, Ladurner R, et al. Response to preoperative chemoembolization correlates with outcome after liver transplantation in patients with hepatocellular carcinoma. Liver Transpl 2007;13(2):272-9.

25. Duffy JP, Vardanian A, Benjamin E, Watson M, Farmer DG, Ghobrial RM, et al. Liver transplantation criteria for hepatocellular carcinoma should be expanded: a 22-year experience with 467 patients at UCLA. Ann Surg 2007; 246(3):502-9.

26. Leung JY, Zhu AX, Gordon FD, Pratt DS, Mithoefer A, Garrigan K, et al. Liver transplantation outcomes for early-stage hepatocellular carcinoma: results of a multicenter study. Liver Transpl 2004;10(11):1343-54.

27. Llovet JM, Schwartz M, Mazzaferro V. Resection and liver transplantation for hepatocellular carcinoma. Semin Liver Dis 2005;25(2):181-200.

28. Mazzaferro V, Chun YS, Poon RT, Schwartz ME, Yao FY, Marsh JW, et al. Liver transplantation for hepatocellular carcinoma. Ann Surg Oncol 2008; 15(4):1001-7.

29. Cillo U, Vitale A, Grigoletto F, Gringeri E, D'Amico F, Valmasoni M, et al. Intention-to-treat analysis of liver transplantation in selected, aggressively treated HCC patients exceeding the Milan criteria. Am J Transplant 2007; 7(4):972-81.

30. Yao FY. Liver transplantation for hepatocellular carcinoma: beyond the Milan criteria. Am J Transplant 2008;8(10):1982-9.

31. Mazzaferro V, Llovet JM, Miceli R, Bhoori S, Schiavo M, Mariani L, et al. Predicting survival after liver transplantation in patients with hepatocellular carcinoma beyond the Milan criteria: a retrospective, exploratory analysis. Lancet Oncol 2009;10(1):35-43.

32. Stieber AC, Marino IR, Iwatsuki S, Starzl TE. Cholangiocarcinoma in sclerosing cholangitis. The role of liver transplantation. Int Surg 1989;74(1):1-3.

33. Goldstein RM, Stone M, Tillery GW, Senzer N, Levy M, Husberg BS, et al. Is liver transplantation indicated for cholangiocarcinoma? Am J Surg 1993; 166(6):768-71.

34. Meyer CG, Penn I, James L. Liver transplantation for cholangiocarcinoma: results in 207 patients. Transplantation 2000;69(8):1633-7.

35. Young AL, Prasad KR, Toogood GJ, Lodge JP. Surgical treatment of hilar cholangiocarcinoma in a new era: comparison among leading Eastern and Western centers, Leeds. J Hepatobiliary Pancreat Surg 2009; [Epub ahead of print].

36. Rea DJ, Heimbach JK, Rosen CB, Haddock MG, Alberts SR, Kremers WK, et al. Liver transplantation with neoadjuvant chemoradiation is more effective than resection for hilar cholangiocarcinoma. Ann Surg 2005;242(3):451-8.

37. Eisenbach C, Merle U, Stremmel W, Encke J. Liver transplantation in HIV-positive patients. Clin Transplant 2009;23(Suppl 21):68-74.

38. Huprikar S. Solid organ transplantation in HIV-infected individuals: an update. Rev Med Virol 2009;19(6):317-23.

39. Broering DC, Topp S, Schaefer U, Fischer L, Gundlach M, Sterneck M, et al. Split liver transplantation and risk to the adult recipient: analysis using matched pairs. J Am Coll Surg 2002;195(5):648-57.

40. Ghobrial RM, Yersiz H, Farmer DG, Amersi F, Goss J, Chen P, et al. Predictors of survival after In vivo split liver transplantation: analysis of 110 consecutive patients. Ann Surg 2000;232(3):312-23.

41. Merion RM, Rush SH, Dykstra DM, Goodrich N, Freeman RB, Jr., Wolfe RA. Predicted lifetimes for adult and pediatric split liver versus adult whole liver transplant recipients. Am J Transplant 2004;4(11):1792-7.

42. Kilic M, Seu P, Stribling RJ, Ghalib R, Goss JA. In situ splitting of the cadaveric liver for two adult recipients. Transplantation 2001;72(11):1853-8.

43. Zamir G, Olthoff KM, Desai N, Markmann JF, Shaked A. Toward further expansion of the organ pool for adult liver recipients: splitting the cadaveric liver into right and left lobes. Transplantation 2002;74(12):1757-61.

44. Bismuth H, Morino M, Castaing D, Gillon MC, Descorps DA, Saliba F, et al. Emergency orthotopic liver transplantation in two patients using one donor liver. Br J Surg 1989;76(7):722-4.

45. Broering DC, Wilms C, Lenk C, Schulte am EJ, Schonherr S, Mueller L, et al. Technical refinements and results in full-right full-left splitting of the deceased donor liver. Ann Surg 2005;242(6):802-12, discussion.

46. Fan ST, Lo CM, Liu CL, Yong BH, Chan JK, Ng IO. Safety of donors in live donor liver transplantation using right lobe grafts. Arch Surg 2000; 135(3):336-40.

47. Northup PG, Berg CL. Living donor liver transplantation: the historical and cultural basis of policy decisions and ongoing ethical questions. Health Policy 2005;72(2):175-85.

48. Surman OS, Cosimi AB, Fukunishi I, Kawaii T, Findley J, Kita Y, et al. Some ethical and psychiatric aspects of right-lobe liver transplantation in the United States and Japan. Psychosomatics 2002;43(5):347-53.

49. Tanaka K, Uemoto S, Honda K, Morimoto T, Tanaka A, Shimabara Y, et al. [Living related liver transplantation]. Nippon Rinsho 1991;49(11):2725-31.

50. Fan ST, Lo CM, Chan KL, Lo R, Saing H, Wei W, et al. Liver transplantation—perspective from Hong Kong. Hepatogastroenterology 1996;43(10):893-7.

51. Lee KU, Kim SB, Kim SH, Lee HJ, Suh KS, Kim ST. Liver transplantation in Seoul National University Hospital. Transplant Proc 2002;34(7):2799-2800.

52. Selzner M, Kashfi A, Cattral MS, Selzner N, McGilvray ID, Greig PD, et al. Live donor liver transplantation in high MELD score recipients. Ann Surg 2010;251(1):153-7.

53. Attia M, Silva MA, Mirza DF. The marginal liver donor—an update. Transpl Int 2008;21(8):713-24.

54. Imber CJ, St Peter SD, Lopez I, Guiver L, Friend PJ. Current practice regarding the use of fatty livers: a trans-Atlantic survey. Liver Transpl 2002; 8(6):545-9.

55. Kievit JK, Oomen AP, Heineman E, Kootstra G. The importance of non-heart-beating donor kidneys in reducing the organ shortage. EDTNA ERCA J 1997; 23(2):11-3.

56. Otero A, Gomez-Gutierrez M, Suarez F, Arnal F, Fernandez-Garcia A, Aguirrezabalaga J, et al. Liver transplantation from Maastricht category 2 non-heart-beating donors. Transplantation 2003;76(7):1068-73.

57. Merion RM, Pelletier SJ, Goodrich N, Englesbe MJ, Delmonico FL. Donation after cardiac death as a strategy to increase deceased donor liver availability. Ann Surg 2006;244(4):555-62.

58. Lee KW, Cameron AM, Maley WR, Segev DL, Montgomery RA. Factors affecting graft survival after adult/child split-liver transplantation: analysis of the UNOS/OPTN data base. Am J Transplant 2008;8(6):1186-96.

59. Muiesan P, Girlanda R, Jassem W, Melendez HV, O'Grady J, Bowles M, et al. Single-center experience with liver transplantation from controlled non-heartbeating donors: a viable source of grafts. Ann Surg 2005;242(5):732-8.

60. Kootstra G, Daemen JH, Oomen AP. Categories of non-heart-beating donors. Transplant Proc 1995;27(5):2893-4.

61. Garcia-Valdecasas JC, Tabet J, Valero R, Taura P, Rull R, Garcia F, et al. Liver conditioning after cardiac arrest: the use of normothermic recirculation in an experimental animal model. Transpl Int 1998;11(6):424-32.

62. Brockmann J, Reddy S, Coussios C, Pigott D, Guirriero D, Hughes D, et al. Normothermic perfusion: a new paradigm for organ preservation. Ann Surg 2009;250(1):1-6.

CHAPTER ■ FIVE

Gallbladder Cancer:
The Rationale for Aggressive Resection

Tim Underwood

BACKGROUND

Gallbladder cancer is the commonest cancer of the biliary tract with a prevalence that varies widely between geographical areas. In the west, gallbladder cancer is a relatively rare disease (US incidence 1-2/100,000) but in northern India the incidence reaches 10.6/100,000, making gallbladder cancer the third commonest cancer after breast and cervical carcinoma in that area.[1,2] Carcinoma of the gallbladder is strongly associated with cholelithiasis (80% of patients with gallbladder cancer will have gallstones) and other factors, such as smoking, female sex, obesity and an isolated large gallbladder polyp (> 10 mm) have all been implicated in the etiology of the disease.[3] The early symptoms of gallbladder cancer include right upper quadrant pain, nausea and anorexia, which are shared by patients with simple cholelithiasis. The non-specific nature of the early symptoms and the propensity of gallbladder cancer towards early dissemination mean that many patients will present late in the course of the disease. The data from large series reflect these problems with overall five-year survivals of no more than 5 to 10%.[4,5] The widespread application of abdominal ultrasonography may lead to the detection of gallbladder polyps and an early gallbladder cancer in some patients. However, the usual mode of diagnosis of gallbladder cancer before late stage symptoms develop is incidentally at the time of laparoscopic cholecystectomy. Since the widespread acceptance of laparoscopic techniques for the management of biliary tract pathology in the early 1990s, the number of laparoscopic cholecystectomies performed each year in the US has risen to over 750,000.[6] Of these cases approximately 5,250 (0.7%) will be found to have gallbladder cancer in the surgical specimen. This may offer the potential to intervene at an earlier stage in the disease process with a theoretical expectation of improved outcome.

Not surprisingly, outcomes are worse as tumor stage at diagnosis increases. Table 5.1 shows the two commonly used staging systems for gallbladder cancer. The five-year survival for stage I patients in the

TABLE 5.1

TNM and American Joint Committee on Cancer Staging of gallbladder cancer. *Adapted from: AJCC Cancer Staging Manual. 6th ed. New York, NY: Springer, 2002;139-44*

TNM Definitions

Primary tumor (T)

- TX: Primary tumor cannot be assessed
- T0: No evidence of primary tumor
- Tis: Carcinoma *in situ*
- T1: Tumor invades lamina propria or muscle layer
  - T1a: Tumor invades lamina propria
  - T1b: Tumor invades the muscle layer
- T2: Tumor invades the perimuscular connective tissue; no extension beyond the serosa or into the liver
- T3: Tumor perforates the serosa (visceral peritoneum) and/or directly invades the liver and/or one other adjacent organ or structure, such as the stomach, duodenum, colon, or pancreas, omentum or extrahepatic bile ducts
- T4: Tumor invades main portal vein or hepatic artery or invades multiple extrahepatic organs or structures

Regional lymph nodes (N)

- NX: Regional lymph nodes cannot be assessed
- N0: No regional lymph node metastasis
- N1: Regional lymph node metastasis

Distant metastasis (M)

- MX: Distant metastasis cannot be assessed
- M0: No distant metastasis
- M1: Distant metastasis

AJCC Stage Groupings

Stage 0	Tis, N0, M0
Stage IA	T1, N0, M0
Stage IB	T2, N0, M0
Stage IIA	T3, N0, M0
Stage IIB	T1, N1, M0/T2, N1, M0/T3, N1, M0
Stage III	T4, any N, M0
Stage IV	Any T, any N, M1

majority of major series is 60 to 70%. Stage II patients can expect a 5-year survival of 30 to 40%, whereas for patients with stage IV disease 5-year survival is 0%.

Surgery offers the only possibility of cure for patients with gallbladder cancer. For patients with early stage disease (Tis and T1), laparoscopic cholecystectomy alone will be curative in 95% of cases.[7,9] Advances in surgery of the liver and biliary tree over recent years have led to the possibility of performing radical resections for gallbladder cancer with curative intent even in very advanced disease. These developments have led to a number of groups presenting data suggesting that radical primary resection and radical re-resection following (laparoscopic) cholecystectomy is feasible, safe and with good medium term outcomes. Unfortunately, the relative rarity of gallbladder cancer means that the majority of published series in the west are retrospective analyses consisting of small numbers of patients treated over relatively long periods of time. Despite these deficiencies, key themes are emerging that should guide the current management of patients presenting with both symptomatic and incidental carcinoma of the gallbladder.

Key Points

- Surgery offers the only possibility of cure for gallbladder cancer.
- Cholecystectomy alone is curative in 95% of patients with Tis and T1a disease.

RADICAL RESECTION IMPROVES SURVIVAL

Interest in the role of radical resection for gallbladder cancer was initiated by reports from Japan suggesting that a survival benefit could be achieved for advanced disease presenting without distant metastasis.[10,15] These studies suggested that an R0 resection was a prerequisite for long-term survival[14] and that this could be achieved by radical local surgery with lymphadenectomy. Surgery for stage III and stage IV disease was, however, associated with an 18% in-hospital mortality.[10] This aggressive strategy has gained popularity in North America with several groups[8,9,16,17] reporting five-year survivals of 35 to 42% following extended resection. In these series, the reported in-hospital mortality rates are less than 5% in keeping with the recent advances in complex hepatobiliary (HPB) surgery. Similar results have been reported from European, Indian and Chinese centers.[18-20] A retrospective analysis of our own data between 1998 and 2008 from a tertiary referral center in the UK has shown an overall 5-year survival of 40%. Median survival increases from 17 months for those patients unsuitable for radical resection to 49 months ($p = 0.05$) with an extended resection (Fig. 5.1). The majority of patients who underwent radical surgery in these series presented with T2 and T3 disease. These patients often cause a dilemma for the inexperienced or infrequent HPB surgeon and have been the subject of much debate in the surgical literature.

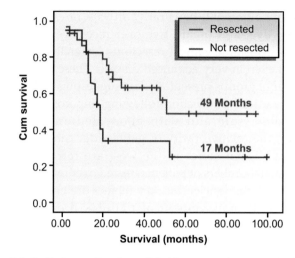

Fig. 5.1: Radical resection for gallbladder cancer improves survival.

Key Point

- Radical surgery improves median survival from 17 to 49 months in suitable patients.

RADICAL SURGERY SHOULD BE CONSIDERED FOR ALL PATIENTS WITH DISEASE STAGES T1B OR GREATER

Consensus exists for the management of T1a disease, which is usually cured by laparoscopic cholecystectomy alone. In bulky T4 disease, radical surgery offers the possibility of tumor clearance, symptom control and sometimes cure. However, a variety of strategies for the management of patients with T2 and T3 disease has been suggested. Some groups limit patients with T2 disease to a simple cholecystectomy unless tumor invasion is greater than 2 mm or lymphovascular invasion in observed in the resected specimen.[21] Others have argued that patients with late stage disease do not derive sufficient benefit from radical surgery, which is associated with significant morbidity and mortality, particularly in asymptomatic patients.[22] Large prospective series have established the safety and efficiency of major liver resection for malignant disease and render these concerns outdated.[23] In the most recent large series, patients with T2 and T3 tumors are observed to derive the maximum benefit from radical resection. Foster et al reviewed 64 patients suffering with gall-bladder cancer at the Roswell Park Cancer Institute between 1972 and 2002.[8] Simple cholecystectomy was the only surgery performed for 25 patients with T2 and T3 disease, whereas 13 patients underwent radical surgery for the same stages of disease. The 5-year survival improved from 16% (95% CI 0-32%) to 62% (95% CI 35-99%) with radical surgery. Similar results were observed by Shih et al for T2 tumors. In this series median survival increased from 6 months to 18 months (p < 0.001) after radical resection.[9] The experience in Southampton is similar with an increase in median survival from 15 to 46 months ($p = 0.03$) after radical surgery for T2 and T3 disease.

The weight of evidence now suggests that patients with T1b disease should be offered radical resection. In the Roswell Park series three patients suffering with T1 disease (one patient with T1a and two with T1b) and were treated with simple cholecystectomy. There was one death at 15 months of a patient with T1b disease with lymphovascular invasion; a finding that may be present in up to 30% of T1b cancers and which is associated with poor outcome.[8,24] Other groups have reported similar findings, with all reported deaths from T1 disease occurring in patients with T1b tumors.[24,25] In particular, the retrospective study performed by Wagholikar et al analyzed two patients with T1a disease and 12 patients with T1b disease. They reported a median overall survival of 42 months with 5 cases of locoregional recurrence and death, all with T1b tumors.[25] Together, the results of multiple studies performed over the last 15 years indicate that radical surgery with curative intent for gallbladder cancer improves survival for T1b, T2, T3 and T4 disease amenable to resection; however, the type and timing of surgery that should be performed and the impact of lymph node positivity and biliary excision require further discussion.

Key Point

- Muscle invasion is associated with poor outcome and patients suffering with T1b disease should be considered for radical resection.

RADICAL RESECTION FOR GALLBLADDER CANCER SHOULD TAKE PLACE IN A SPECIALIST CENTER

The surgeon making an incidental finding of gallbladder cancer at cholecystectomy faces a decision to perform radical surgery during the same operation or complete the cholecystectomy and wait for formal histological confirmation of gallbladder carcinoma before contemplating a radical resection. This decision may be straightforward in patients unfit for major liver resection but for young patients without significant comorbidity, it is tempting to convert to open operation in an attempt to perform an R0 resection. Indeed, this approach is advocated by some if both the diagnosis and stage have been established on frozen section and provided there is no evidence of intraperitoneal dissemination on exploratory laparoscopy.[26] This strategy has a theoretical advantage as gallbladder cancer is an aggressive disease and an interval between diagnosis and radical excision may increase the likelihood of dissemination. Proponents of this approach stress that the surgeon should have the experience and expertise to perform a major hepatobiliary resection. If these skills are not available, patients diagnosed with gallbladder cancer during or after laparoscopic cholecystectomy should be referred to a specialist HPB unit for further treatment. Fortunately, the outcomes for these patients do not seem to differ from those undergoing primary resection. In the series from Johns Hopkins there was no difference in the 5-year survival of patients who had their potentially curative resection performed at initial surgery or during a second procedure,[9] a finding that is supported by other published series.[8,16,26,27] It is clear that gallbladder cancer exhibits a propensity for seeding into laparoscopic port sites[28-31] and care should be taken at the first operation to extract an intact (non-perforated) gallbladder in an impervious retrieval bag. The risks of port site metastasis lead most major centers to advocate port site excision at the time of radical surgery. A modern strategy for the management of suspected gallbladder cancer consists of early referral to a specialist HPB center with excellent imaging facilities to facilitate planned liver resection. For a patient with unsuspected gallbladder cancer found at surgery in a non-specialist centre the procedure should be abandoned and urgent referral made to the local HPB unit. A similar patient being treated within the regional center may be converted to gallbladder fossa resection with frozen section, allowing the possibility of lymphadenectomy and biliary resection with curative intent, depending on the extent of disease.

Key Points

- Radical surgery should take place in a specialist center either as the primary operation or as a delayed procedure following cholecystectomy at another hospital.
- Referral to a specialist center following the diagnosis of incidental gallbladder cancer is not associated with worse outcome.

WHAT SURGERY TO PERFORM?

The rationale for radical surgery in gallbladder cancer is established but debate remains regarding the extent and nature of the resection that is required. To some degree this is determined by the stage of the disease at diagnosis. A multivisceral resection may be considered in a young, fit patient if preoperative staging suggests that an R0 resection will be possible. In addition, aggressive surgery for bulky T4 disease has been shown to prolong survival and provide excellent symptom control.[10-13] In most instances, this kind of surgery will not be required, especially for those patients presenting with incidental tumors. After cholecystectomy, residual tumor will be found in the liver at re-operation in 34 to 89% of cases[32,33] and under these circumstances most groups agree that radical surgery involves resection of the gallbladder fossa (either a non-anatomical or anatomical segment IVb/V resection) with locoregional lymphadenectomy +/- resection of the extrahepatic biliary ducts.[2,8-10,19,24,26] In 10 years at Southampton, radical surgery has given excellent results, with over 80% of resections being an anatomical segment IVb/V excision + lymphadenectomy or formal right hemihepatectomy + lymphadenectomy. In this series, no patient with T2 disease was found to have residual hepatic disease but all patients with T3 tumors did have residual disease (55% of those undergoing radical re-resection).

The extent of lymphadenectomy to perform is a topic of keen debate. It is clear that gallbladder cancer spreads readily to the local lymphatics, and lymph node metastases have been observed in up to 46% of patients with T2 disease;[34] but this does not take place in every case. Kondo et al has described a classification of gallbladder cancer based on six common types of presentation, including a sub-type where lymphatic spread occurs early despite the primary tumor, remaining small and confined to the gallbladder.[35] Furthermore, Shibata et al suggest that the presence of lymphatic invasion should be used to identify those patients who require radical resection after the discovery of T1b-T3 tumors in laparoscopic cholecystectomy specimens.[36] Shimada et al addressed the relationship between lymph node involvement and survival after radical resection in 41 patients over an 11-year period. When reviewed according to site, the rate of locoregional lymph node involvement was 41.5% in pericholedochal lymph nodes, 22.0% in the lymph nodes around the common hepatic artery and the portal vein, 36.6% in the posterior pancreaticoduodenal lymph nodes, 28% in the celiac lymph nodes, 19% in the superior mesenteric artery lymph nodes and 26% in the aortocaval/para-aortic lymph nodes.[37] Patients with severe hepatoduodenal ligament invasion were noted to have high rates of para-aortic lymph node involvement. When this cohort was analyzed by T stage, the 5-year survival rate for pT2 disease was 72.7% in patients with pN0+ pN1+ positive posterior pancreaticoduodenal lymph nodes or positive lymph nodes around the common hepatic artery and nil in the patients with positive celiac, superior mesenteric artery (SMA) and para-aortic lymph nodes ($p < 0.05$). The consensus of opinion suggests that patients with T1a-T3 N1 disease may achieve long-term survival with radical resection (some groups suggest that this applies for T4 disease also) if the positive nodes are confined to the hepato-duodenal ligament, but the finding of positive nodes in more distant nodal stations is associated with very poor outcomes irrespective of T stage. Recent North American series question this statement, as at least one patient is alive 75 months after radical surgery for distant nodal disease[8] and lymphadenectomy was found to be predictive of improved outcome on multivariate analysis.[9]

There is little evidence to support routine excision of the extra-hepatic biliary tree during surgery for gallbladder cancer unless there is a positive cystic duct margin on frozen section or excision is necessary for the completion of an R0 resection. In their review of 107 patients with gallbladder cancer, Shih et al found no evidence of survival benefit from biliary excision over and above that achieved by radical resection for T2 disease.

Key Points

- R0 resection with lymphadenectomy improves survival.
- Routine resection of the extra-hepatic biliary tree is not supported by current evidence.

SUMMARY

Gallbladder cancer is an aggressive malignancy and the majority of patients will be unsuitable for curative resection at the time of diagnosis. The greater uptake of laparoscopic cholecystectomy for gallstone disease has increased the likelihood of discovering gallbladder cancer incidentally and possibly at an earlier stage. Improvements in mortality and morbidity rates following major hepatobiliary procedures have meant that patients that would formerly have been assessed as unsuitable for radical resection have been offered a potential cure. The initial enthusiasm for radical resection for gallbladder cancer in Japan has been repeated in several centers in North America and Europe. The results of retrospective series from these institutions over the last 15 years are encouraging. Despite the lack of randomized controlled trials (due to the rarity of the disease) we can be confident that surgery offers the only possibility of cure for gallbladder cancer.

Patients suffering with T1a disease after laparoscopic cholecystectomy will have been cured by their initial operation. For patients with higher stage disease, radical resection is indicated if the possibility of an R0 resection exists on preoperative staging. The extent of surgery will be determined by the extent of disease. Most groups advocate a minimum of non-anatomical gallbladder fossa resection with portal lymphadenectomy for incidental tumors, performed at the time of first operation only if there is adequate local expertise. Despite the theoretical risk of tumor progression if radical surgery is delayed this fear is not born out in any large series. If gallbladder cancer is discovered postoperatively after cholecystectomy, patients should be referred to a specialized HPB unit for consideration of radical reoperation. In such centers extended hepatic resections with multiple field lymphadenectomy can achieve complete tumor excision. Under these circumstances the once miserable 5-year survival rates of 5% have risen to over 40%.

REFERENCES

1. Misra MC, Guleria S. Management of cancer gallbladder found as a surprise on a resected gallbladder specimen. J Surg Oncol 2006;93(8):690-8.
2. Fong Y, Malhotra S. Gallbladder cancer: recent advances and current guidelines for surgical therapy. Adv Surg 2001;35:1-20.
3. Scott TE, Carroll M, Cogliano FD, Smith BF, Lamorte WW. A case-control assessment of risk factors for gallbladder carcinoma. Dig Dis Sci 1999; 44(8):1619-25.

4. Cubertafond P, Gainant A, Cucchiaro G. Surgical treatment of 724 carcinomas of the gallbladder. Results of the French Surgical Association Survey. Ann Surg 1994;219(3):275-80.

5. Piehler JM, Crichlow RW. Primary carcinoma of the gallbladder. Surg Gynecol Obstet 1978;147(6):929-42.

6. Shaffer EA. Epidemiology and risk factors for gallstone disease: has the paradigm changed in the 21st century? Curr Gastroenterol Rep 2005;7(2): 132-40.

7. Yamaguchi K, Tsuneyoshi M. Subclinical gallbladder carcinoma. Am J Surg 1992;163(4):382-6.

8. Foster JM, Hoshi H, Gibbs JF, Iyer R, Javle M, Chu Q, et al. Gallbladder cancer: Defining the indications for primary radical resection and radical re-resection. Ann Surg Oncol 2007;14(2):833-40.

9. Shih SP, Schulick RD, Cameron JL, Lillemoe KD, Pitt HA, Choti MA, et al. Gallbladder cancer: the role of laparoscopy and radical resection. Ann Surg 2007;245(6):893-901.

10. Kondo S, Nimura Y, Hayakawa N, Kamiya J, Nagino M, Uesaka K. Extensive surgery for carcinoma of the gallbladder. Br J Surg 2002;89(2):179-84.

11. Kondo S, Nimura Y, Kamiya J, Nagino M, Kanai M, Uesaka K, et al. Five-year survivors after aggressive surgery for stage IV gallbladder cancer. J Hepatobiliary Pancreat Surg 2001;8(6):511-7.

12. Kondo S, Nimura Y, Kamiya J, Nagino M, Kanai M, Uesaka K, et al. Factors influencing postoperative hospital mortality and long-term survival after radical resection for stage IV gallbladder carcinoma. World J Surg 2003; 27(3):272-7.

13. Shirai Y, Ohtani T, Tsukada K, Hatakeyama K. Radical surgery is justified for locally advanced gallbladder carcinoma if complete resection is feasible. Am J Gastroenterol 1997;92(1):181-2.

14. Shirai Y, Yoshida K, Tsukada K, Muto T, Watanabe H. Radical surgery for gallbladder carcinoma. Long-term results. Ann Surg 1992;216(5):565-8.

15. Todoroki T, Kawamoto T, Takahashi H, Takada Y, Koike N, Otsuka M, et al. Treatment of gallbladder cancer by radical resection. Br J Surg 1999; 86(5):622-7.

16. Fong Y, Jarnagin W, Blumgart LH. Gallbladder cancer: comparison of patients presenting initially for definitive operation with those presenting after prior noncurative intervention. Ann Surg 2000;232(4):557-69.

17. Dixon E, Vollmer CM, Jr., Sahajpal A, Cattral M, Grant D, Doig C, et al. An aggressive surgical approach leads to improved survival in patients with gallbladder cancer: a 12-year study at a North American Center. Ann Surg 2005;241(3):385-94.

18. Liang JW, Dong SX, Zhou ZX, Tian YT, Zhao DB, Wang CF, et al. Surgical management for carcinoma of the gallbladder: a single-institution experience in 25 years. Chin Med J (Engl) 2008;121(19):1900-5.

19. Misra S, Chaturvedi A, Misra NC. Gallbladder cancer. Curr Treat Options Gastroenterol 2006;9(2):95-106.

20. Principe A, Del Gaudio M, Ercolani G, Golfieri R, Cucchetti A, Pinna AD. Radical surgery for gallbladder carcinoma: possibilities of survival. Hepatogastroenterology 2006;53(71):660-4.

21. Wakai T, Shirai Y, Yokoyama N, Ajioka Y, Watanabe H, Hatakeyama K. Depth of subserosal invasion predicts long-term survival after resection in patients with T2 gallbladder carcinoma. Ann Surg Oncol 2003;10(4):447-54.

22. Oertli D, Herzog U, Tondelli P. Primary carcinoma of the gallbladder: operative experience during a 16 years period. Eur J Surg 1993;159(8):415-20.

23. Simillis C, Constantinides VA, Tekkis PP, Darzi A, Lovegrove R, Jiao L, et al. Laparoscopic versus open hepatic resections for benign and malignant neoplasms—a meta-analysis. Surgery 2007;141(2):203-11.

24. Ouchi K, Suzuki M, Tominaga T, Saijo S, Matsuno S. Survival after surgery for cancer of the gallbladder. Br J Surg 1994;81(11):1655-7.

25. Wagholikar GD, Behari A, Krishnani N, Kumar A, Sikora SS, Saxena R, et al. Early gallbladder cancer. J Am Coll Surg 2002;194(2):137-41.

26. Yeh CN, Jan YY, Chen MF. Management of unsuspected gallbladder carcinoma discovered during or following laparoscopic cholecystectomy. Am Surg 2004;70(3):256-8.

27. Lohe F, Meimarakis G, Schauer C, Angele M, Jauch KW, Schauer RJ. The time of diagnosis impacts surgical management but not the outcome of patients with gallbladder carcinoma. Eur J Med Res 2009;14(8):345-51.

28. Clair DG, Lautz DB, Brooks DC. Rapid development of umbilical metastases after laparoscopic cholecystectomy for unsuspected gallbladder carcinoma. Surgery 1993;113(3):355-8.

29. Drouard F, Delamarre J, Capron JP. Cutaneous seeding of gallbladder cancer after laparoscopic cholecystectomy. N Engl J Med 1991;325(18):1316.

30. Fong Y, Brennan MF, Turnbull A, Colt DG, Blumgart LH. Gallbladder cancer discovered during laparoscopic surgery. Potential for iatrogenic tumour dissemination. Arch Surg 1993;128(9):1054-6.

31. Winston CB, Chen JW, Fong Y, Schwartz LH, Panicek DM. Recurrent gallbladder carcinoma along laparoscopic cholecystectomy port tracks: CT demonstration. Radiology 1999;212(2):439-44.

32. Ogura Y, Mizumoto R, Isaji S, Kusuda T, Matsuda S, Tabata M. Radical operations for carcinoma of the gallbladder: present status in Japan. World J Surg 1991;15(3):337-43.

33. Wanebo HJ, Vezeridis MP. Carcinoma of the gallbladder. J Surg Oncol Suppl 1993;3:134-9.

34. Bartlett DL, Fong Y, Fortner JG, Brennan MF, Blumgart LH. Long-term results after resection for gallbladder cancer. Implications for staging and management. Ann Surg 1996;224(5):639-46.

35. Kondo S, Nimura Y, Kamiya J, Nagino M, Kanai M, Uesaka K, et al. Mode of tumour spread and surgical strategy in gallbladder carcinoma. Langenbecks Arch Surg 2002;387(5-6):222-8.

36. Shibata K, Uchida H, Iwaki K, Kai S, Ohta M, Kitano S. Lymphatic invasion: an important prognostic factor for stages T1b-T3 gallbladder cancer and an indication for additional radical resection of incidental gallbladder cancer. World J Surg 2009;33(5):1035-41.

37. Shimada H, Endo I, Togo S, Nakano A, Izumi T, Nakagawara G. The role of lymph node dissection in the treatment of gallbladder carcinoma. Cancer 1997;79(5):892-9.

CHAPTER SIX

Surgery for Chronic Pancreatitis

Colin D Johnson

Chronic pancreatitis is an incurable condition with a spectrum of severity from mild to very severe. Symptoms may have an adverse effect on the quality of life and complications may require admission to hospital and may be life threatening. The usual clinical presentation is with upper abdominal pain, followed after a variable period of time by pancreatic exocrine insufficiency and/or diabetes mellitus. Strong analgesia is required to deal with the debilitating pain and the metabolic and nutritional disturbances may lead to severe cachexia and increased susceptibility to infection.

Four main etiological groups are recognized. Alcohol related and idiopathic pancreatitis account for up to 90% of cases in western series and obstruction of the main pancreatic duct by a tumor or stricture accounts for the remainder. These diagnoses are found usually in middle-aged or older patients. Tropical pancreatitis is seen in several countries of Asia, the Indian subcontinent and Africa: it is best described in south India but it seems to be declining in incidence.[1] The causative mechanism is unknown, but may reflect an interaction of genetic factors with malnutrition in childhood or intrauterine life. Onset is often in childhood and advanced disease is seen in patients aged 15-30: cancer may develop at a young age.

There are minor differences in clinical features and morphology in these diagnostic groups but the principles of treatment are the same irrespective of etiology.

Medical treatment is largely supportive. Pain is usually managed with opioid analgesics, with the addition of adjuvant analgesics if required. Pancreatic enzyme insufficiency responds to enzyme supplements taken with every meal and diabetes usually requires insulin therapy.

Complications of chronic pancreatitis include stricture of the lower common bile duct with obstructive jaundice, duodenal fibrosis with gastric outlet obstruction and pancreatic pseudocyst. The indications for surgical treatment in chronic pancreatitis are similar to those of surgical treatment in other benign chronic conditions: that is; failure of medical

TABLE 6.1

Indications for operation and treatment options

Pain	Pancreatic drainage Resection Nerve block - CPB or TS

Complications
— Obstructive jaundice
 	
— Duodenal obstruction/ulceration
— Pseudocyst
	Drainage
	— Choloedochojejunostomy
	   or resection
	— Gastrojejunostomy or resection
	— Endoscopic or surgical
	   drainage, pancreatic resection

management (particularly for pain) and the treatment of complications as shown in Table 6.1. In this chapter, I will not consider the management of pseudocyst.

SURGICAL OPTIONS FOR PAIN RELIEF

Surgery can offer three main categories of procedure for the relief of pain. Nerve ablation procedures are designed to interrupt the pain pathways from the pancreas; they relieve symptoms without addressing the underlying disease. Decompression/resection of pancreatic tissue is designed to relieve pancreatic duct obstruction, reduce pancreatic tissue pressure and thereby stabilize the disease and relieve symptoms. Formal pancreatic resection removes the diseased gland, which in theory should prevent further symptoms and complications.

Nerve Ablation Procedures

Painful sensation from the pancreas is carried to the central nervous system in the splanchnic nerves. From the pancreas afferent fibers traverse the celiac plexus and then condense into the splanchnic nerves, which pass through the diaphragm close to the vertebral bodies and continue in the chest to the thoracic sympathetic chain. Ablation procedures designed to interrupt these pathways include the injection of sclerosant into the celiac plexus or into the subdiaphragmatic splanchnic nerves by either percutaneous or endoscopic approaches, as well as surgical ablation of the splanchnic nerves as they traverse the diaphragm or within the chest. This latter approach has been adapted in recent years for a thoracoscopic approach in which all of the splanchnic nerves can be identified and destroyed bilaterally as they approach the sympathetic chains.

Experience of these different approaches[2-6] gives broadly similar results as shown in Table 6.2. Initial response is usually good (>80%) but recurrence of symptoms is usually seen after 6-24 months. The mechanism

TABLE 6.2

Late outcome of nerve ablation procedures in chronic pancreatitis

	% with pain relief	Duration of follow-up
Andren-Sandberg and Ihse[2,3]	93	13 months
	50	43 months
Davis[4]	83	Immediate
	63	1 year
Buscher[5]	52	1 year
	38	2 years
	28	4 years
Baghdadi[6] (systematic review)	90	6 months
	75	1 year
	49	15 months

of recurrence is unclear, but may involve recruitment of afferent vagal fibers, nerve regeneration or extension of the inflammatory process to non-denervated areas.

In surgical practice, the use of nerve ablation procedures is relatively restricted. There may be a role for nerve ablation in patients unfit for laparotomy or as a mean to delay the requirement for surgery. However, in a disease, which affects predominantly young adults and runs a chronic course, recurrence of symptoms is usual and delay in the surgery may adversely affect the eventual functional outcome.

Key Point

- Nerve ablation by celiac plexus block or splanchnicotomy can relieve pain, but the effect is usually short-lived.

Decompression/Resection Procedures

A large numbers of different procedures have been described to deal with the abnormal pancreas. When the main pancreatic duct is extensively dilated, it is tempting to suppose that a duct drainage procedure should relieve symptoms, particularly if there is a dominant stricture close to the ampulla. Reber and colleagues described a compartment syndrome of the pancreas, in which intraductal pressures and parenchymal pressures are elevated in chronic pancreatitis. They demonstrated experimentally that incision of the pancreas for pancreaticojejunostomy produced a similar effect to fasciotomy with reduction of tissue pressures.[7]

These experimental studies suggest that pancreatic decompression may be of benefit even in cases of chronic pancreatitis without pancreatic duct dilatation. The rationale for decompression is that relief of the "compartment syndrome", which improves blood flow in the stimulated pancreas and avoids the painful response to stimulation that characterizes this disease.

Standard pancreaticojejunostomy is relatively straightforward when there is duct dilatation. However, when the pancreatic duct is small it may be difficult to achieve a satisfactory anastomosis by simple incision into the duct. Izbicki and colleagues[8] have described a V-shaped longitudinal resection of the pancreatic body, which leaves a gutter-shaped remnant suitable for pancreatic jejunal anastomosis. With this technique, it is possible to decompress the body of pancreas even in the absence of duct dilatation.

In many patients, the main focus of inflammation is within the head of the pancreas. Two similar procedures have been described to deal with this inflammatory mass while preserving the duodenum. In 1987 Frey[9] described a technique for the extension of pancreaticojejunostomy into the pancreatic head. When the duct in this area was inaccessible or small, he created a space within the head to allow anastomosis of jejunum to the decompressed pancreatic remnant by coring out a central portion of the head of pancreas. This procedure removes a limited amount of pancreatic tissue and therefore minimizes the postoperative change in pancreatic exocrine and endocrine function, but it does not deal with the potential involvement of the bile duct in the inflammatory process and is therefore not sufficient for patients with low bile duct obstruction.

In 1985, Beger[10] had described a large resection of the pancreatic head, involving division of the pancreatic neck and excision of all pancreatic tissue apart from the posterior capsule and a rim of pancreatic tissue on the medial wall of the duodenum, covering the pancreaticoduodenal arcade. This leaves a bowl shaped cavity, which can be anastomosed to the small bowel, after drainage of the left pancreas by pancreatico-jejunostomy. Although it is a resection of the pancreatic head, its effect is to decompress the residual pancreas provided there are no strictures in the main pancreatic duct. If strictures are found, the operation can be extended to include lateral pancreaticojejunostomy of the body and tail.

Buchler described a combination of these two procedures, suitable when the plane between the pancreas and the mesenteric vein is obscured by fibrosis or contains dilated collateral veins. It is possible to omit the step of division of the neck, while ensuring almost complete removal of the head.[10]

When all of these procedures are considered together, it becomes apparent that they constitute a spectrum of drainage/resection in which the aim of effective pancreatic decompression is achieved throughout the whole pancreas (Figs 6.1A to D). The choice of procedure to achieve this aim can be tailored to the extent of disease and the morphological features encountered in each case.

An advantage of the Beger procedure is that bile duct obstruction by pancreatic inflammation and fibrosis can be effectively prevented by removal of pancreatic tissue along one side of the duct. The duct is then easily drained into the pancreatic cavity to give good long-term relief or prevention of jaundice.

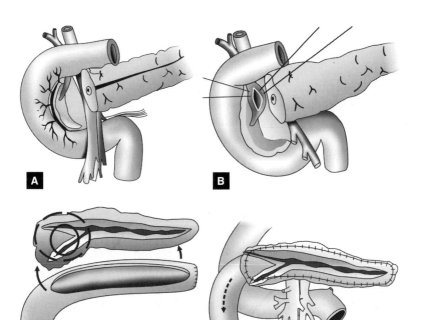

Figs 6.1A to D: The spectrum of drainage/resection procedures. In the Beger operation, almost all the pancreatic head is excised (A). The common bile duct may be opened into the resection cavity for long-term drainage (B). After resection of the head by Beger (dashed line) or Frey (solid line) the pancreatic duct may be opened along its length for drainage of the body (C). The end results of Beger, Frey and lateral pancreatico-jejunostomy are very similar (D). (Figures A and B[9]).

Key Point

- Decompression of the pancreas spares a ranged of procedures from lateral pancreaticojejunostomy to resection of the pancreatic head.

Formal Pancreatic Resection

Occasionally, formal resection may be the best option for surgical treatment of chronic pancreatitis. In a patient, who has had previous pancreatitis or pancreatic trauma, leading to stricture of the pancreatic duct with chronic obstructive pancreatitis to the left of the stricture, left pancreatectomy will be curative. This may be achieved with splenic preservation.[11] However, these cases are rare and the operation should only be undertaken when the head of pancreas is normal. If the chronic pancreatitis affects the whole gland, even when there is predominantly left-sided duct dilatation, a drainage/resection procedure is usually the better option.

In some patients with a mass in the head of pancreas, it may not be possible to exclude with certainty a pancreatic cancer. In these cases, a formal pancreaticoduodenectomy with or without pylorus preservation will remove the inflammatory focus and provide adequate material for accurate histological diagnosis. As described below, pancreaticoduodenectomy gives long-term results for symptom relief in chronic pancreatitis equivalent to the organ sparing drainage/resection procedures. So, it is the appropriate choice of operation when there is a diagnostic doubt.

TIMING OF SURGERY

The appropriate timing of surgical intervention is a matter of judgement. The main indication is for the relief of pain, which cannot be controlled by medical means. Severe continuous pain or repeated exacerbations, which prevent the patient from working or require frequent admissions to hospital despite maximal medical treatment, clearly require a surgical approach. On the other hand, patients with mild pain usually controlled by nonopioid treatments, who continue to pursue their normal activities will be understandably reluctant to undergo surgical treatment and in these cases it is probably unnecessary. In between these extremes, many patients are managed by protracted medical treatment, with frequent interruptions of their life by exacerbations of the disease. It is unfortunately still often the case that patients who might benefit from surgery are not referred for a specialist opinion at an appropriate time. Not only does surgery offer about 80% chance of good pain relief (and cessation or substantial reduction in opioid use as described below), but there is some evidence that early surgery may help to preserve and even improve pancreatic function.

In a combined prospective cohort study and randomized trial Nealon and Thompson[12] demonstrated that patients with early painful chronic pancreatitis with duct dilatation offered surgery were much less likely to progress to severe pancreatic insufficiency and to have a good outcome from surgery than those who were initially offered medical treatment only (Table 6.3).

It is difficult to confirm with objective data but it remains a widely held view amongst pancreatic surgeons that persistence of medical treatment with several years of regular opioid use is associated with a poor outcome, compared with the better outcome observed after surgery performed earlier in the disease. This reflects the difficulty of stopping treatment with opioids after many years and the associated tendency of the patients to require opioid treatment for any abdominal sensation, which they perceive as pain.

Key Point

- Easily operation effectively prevents loss of function in patients with dilated pancreatic duct.

TABLE 6.3

Late outcome (numbers with mild or moderate pancreatitis) in a combined cohort study/ randomized trial of surgery vs no operation in patients with mild or moderate chronic pancreatitis and duct dilation at study entry (Nealon and Thompson[12])

	Initial evaluation	Follow-up
Cohort study		
Operated	47/47	41/47 (87%)
Non-operated	36/36	8/36 (22%)
Randomized trial		
Operated	9/9	7/9 (78%)
Non-operated	8/8	2/8 (25%)

SURGICAL DRAINAGE OR ENDOSCOPIC TREATMENT FOR DUCT OBSTRUCTION

Endoscopic therapy can achieve temporary duct drainage in patients with a stricture close to the ampulla, by insertion of a stent or in whom there is a stone causing obstruction of the main pancreatic duct within the head. Such treatment can achieve 86 to 95% immediate pain relief but longer term results are disappointing with approximately half the patients experiencing recurrence of pain.[13]

Two randomized trials have evaluated the medium-term results of endoscopic versus surgical therapy in patients with chronic pancreatitis. In the first study by Dite et al[14] on 140 patients with painful obstructive chronic pancreatitis, 72 were randomized to either endoscopic or surgical treatment ($n = 36$ in each group), with the remaining 68 opting for either surgical ($n = 40$) or endoscopic treatment ($n = 28$). All 140 patients had obstructive chronic pancreatitis with a dilated main pancreatic duct, strictures and/or stones predominantly in the pancreatic head or body and significant pain refractory to conservative management. In the endoscopy group ($n = 64$), pancreatic sphincterotomy was performed in all patients and pancreatic stents were placed in 33 (52%). Stone extraction was attempted in 15 patients (23%). The procedure was technically successful in 62 of 64 patients (97%) with an overall post-endoscopic retrograde cholangiopancreatography (ERCP) complication rate of 8%. The mean duration of stenting was 16 months with an average of six stent exchanges per patient. There was no surgical intervention or treatment-associated mortality. In the surgical group ($n = 76$), 61 (80%) underwent resection, including duodenum-preserving pancreatic head resection ($n = 33$), pancreaticoduodenectomy ($n = 23$), distal pancreatectomy ($n = 5$) and pancreaticojejunostomy ($n = 15$). Postoperative complications occurred in 8%. There was no treatment-related mortality. At one year pain relief was similar in the endoscopic and surgical groups. However, at 5 years follow-up, significantly more patients in the surgical group reported complete absence of pain. In addition, there was a significantly greater improvement in body weight in the surgical groups compared to the endoscopic groups.

The second trial[15] was terminated early by the safety committee due to significant differences in outcome in the patients randomized to endoscopic ($n = 19$) or surgical ($n = 20$) drainage. In the endoscopic group, 16/19 patients underwent external shock wave lithotripsy (ESWL) followed by an endoscopic procedure (stent insertion in 16/19, balloon dilatation in 15/19), with insertion of cumulative stents as required. A median of five (range 1–11) therapeutic procedures was performed and the median period of stenting was 27 weeks. Minor complications occurred in 58% of patients and there was one death. In four of the 19 patients, surgical drainage was subsequently performed for intractable abdominal pain. In the surgical group, 18/20 patients underwent lateral pancreatojejunostomy with one patient each undergoing pancreaticoduodenectomy or a Frey procedure (for stone extraction). Minor complications occurred in 35%. The median number of therapeutic procedures was significantly higher in the endoscopic group compared to that of the surgical group (8:3, $p < 0.001$). The technical success rates were 53% and 100% for endoscopic and surgical procedures, respectively ($p < 0.001$). Complete or partial pain relief was achieved at the end of the two-year follow-up among 32% of the endoscopic group and 75% of the surgical group ($p = 0.007$). In addition, the quality of life score for physical health was significantly lower in the endoscopic group compared to the surgical group ($p = 0.003$).

These studies show that when there is evidence of ductal obstruction, surgery gives better long-term symptom relief than endoscopic procedures in chronic pancreatitis. Endoscopic therapy may be able to delay the need for surgery but often results only in additional procedures and a longer duration of preoperative opioid therapy. Some form of surgical resection remains the only definitive option for the majority of patients who do not have duct dilatation.

Key Point

- Trial evidence shows that endoscopy for duct obstruction may delay surgery, but operation has greater long-term success.

CHOICE OF SURGICAL PROCEDURE

A number of randomized controlled trials of surgery for chronic pancreatitis help us to decide, which operation is appropriate. Although the numbers included in individual studies are small, these trials are well designed and benefit from being single center studies in high volume institutions. This means the patient groups in each study are relatively uniform, that the recruitment was achieved in a relatively short time and

that long-term follow-up is possible.

TABLE 6.4

Early results from randomized trials of surgical procedures in chronic pancreatitis. LPJ/ LPHE: Lateral pancreaticojejunostomy with localized pancreatic head excision; PP: pylorus preserving Whipple operation

	Follow-up	Operation	n	Surgical compli- cations	Reduced pain or pain free	QoL	Wt gain
Izbicki	*5y (1-10)*	LPJ/LPHE	31		94%	86	82%
		PPW	30	19%	95%	57	40%
Buchler	6 months	Beger	20	15%	75%		88%
		PPW	20	20%	40%		67%
Farkas	*1-3 y*	LPJ/LPHE	20	0	85%		7.8 kg
		PPW	20	40%	90%		3.2 kg

By contrast, the long-term outcome in studies reporting non-specialist practice is heavily dependent on the variations in choice of procedure, which may affect outcome. Despite the drawbacks of such studies,[16] the results are reasonably consistent, suggesting that 70 to 80% of patients will be free of opioids in long-term follow-up, that about two thirds of patients will require no analgesia and that modest weight gain after surgery is to be expected.[17,18]

The majority of patients with chronic pancreatitis do not have a dilated pancreatic duct and therefore require some form of resection surgery. It is now clear that this can be achieved with preservation of adjacent organs using the procedures described by Beger[10] in 1985 and Frey[9] in 1987. Preservation of the gastroduodenal axis is said to maximize the potential for normal nutritional intake and may help to maintain normal glucose homeostasis, although the progression to diabetes is largely determined by the severity of the chronic pancreatitis throughout the remaining pancreatic tissue.

Three studies[19-21] have compared different surgical procedures (Table 6.4). In Izbicki's hands, a pancreatic decompression by extended Frey procedure and a pylorus preserving Whipple operation gave very similar high numbers of patients with reduced pain postoperatively.[21] Weight gain during early follow-up (mean 5 years) was seen in 82% of the decompression patients compared with only 40% of the Whipple's patients. Farkas[20] with a 1-3 year follow-up found similar advantage of greater weight gain and very high proportion of patients pain free. Buchler[19] compared the Beger procedure with a pylorus preserving Whipple operation and found a much lower proportion of patients pain free and again more patients showing weight gain at six month follow-up after the Whipple operation. In that study, the Beger operation was associated with 80% return to work at six months compared with only 67% after Whipple operation.

The late outcome after decompression/resection procedures or formal pylorus preserving Whipple operation was very similar in three studies. All procedures provide adequate pain relief and quality of life after long-term follow-up with no differences in exocrine and endocrine function.[22-24] In view of the usually shorter operating time and the better short-term results after decompression/resection procedures, these are generally preferred for the relief of pain in chronic pancreatitis.

An important technical point when operating for chronic pancreatitis is to ensure adequate decompression or drainage of the bile duct. A disadvantage of the Frey procedure is that the bile duct is not exposed and as a result recurrence of obstructive jaundice may be more frequent after this operation. During the Beger procedure the common bile duct should be exposed in the posterior wall of the pancreatic cavity. It is possible to decompress the bile duct along its intrapancreatic length, but it is perhaps simpler and more certain to prevent recurrent jaundice by opening the duct and creating an anastomosis between it and the pancreatic cavity. This ensures biliary drainage into the same Roux loop that is draining the residual pancreas.

Adequate excision of the pancreatic head during the Beger procedure usually relieves fibrotic obstruction of the duodenum, which is freed from its enveloping and restricting peripancreatic fibrosis. It is extremely unusual that gastric outlet obstruction cannot be relieved in this way but in such cases a formal pancreaticoduodenectomy will solve the problem.

Key Points

- Pain relief is achieved in the long term for 70-80% of patients who have surgery.
- Organ sparing resection has better short-term results than pancreatico-duodenectomy.

CONCLUSION

Surgical procedures for relief of pain in chronic pancreatitis are more likely to be effective than various endoscopic techniques. Patients without pancreatic duct dilatation (the majority in most series) are not suitable for endoscopic therapy. The operation should be tailored to the individual patient and pancreatic morphology. The aim should be to adequately decompress the whole pancreas. If the pancreatic duct is dilated this aim can be achieved by lateral pancreaticojejunostomy. Often however, there is a mass of inflammatory tissue in the head of the pancreas and this must be resected.

Resection of the pancreatic head can be performed without resection of the duodenum by either the Beger or Frey procedure. The remaining body of pancreas should be adequately drained, by lateral pancreatico-jejunostomy if there is stricturing in the main pancreatic duct.

In the presence of obstructive jaundice, it is imperative to drain the common bile duct during this procedure. It is a wise precaution in any case to ensure that progressive pancreatitis will not lead subsequently to obstructive jaundice by fibrosis around the bile duct as it traverses the pancreatic remnant. Exposure of the common duct and drainage into the cavity, created by excision of the head, is usually appropriate and provides effective long-term biliary drainage.

Gastric outlet obstruction is usually relieved by an adequate head resection even with preservation of the duodenum. However, in cases where there is concern about duodenal involvement, or where the differential diagnosis between chronic pancreatitis and pancreatic cancer is in doubt, the surgeon can perform a formal pancreaticoduodenectomy. This has a higher immediate complication rate and less good short- to medium-term results than the drainage/resection procedures but in the long-term (up to 10 years and more) outcomes are similar.

REFERENCES

1. Balakrishnan V, Unnikrishnan AG, Thomas V, Choudhuri G, Veeraraju P, Singh SP, et al. Chronic pancreatitis: A prospective nationwide study of 1,086 subjects from India. JOP 2008;9(5):593-600.
2. Ihse I, Zoucas E, Gyllstedt E, Lillo-Gil R, Andren-Sandberg A. Bilateral thoracoscopic splanchnicectomy: effects on pancreatic pain and function. Ann Surg 1999;230(6):785-90.
3. Andren-Sandberg A, Zoucas E, Lillo-Gil R, Gyllstedt E, Ihse I. Thoracoscopic Splanchnicectomy for Chronic, Severe Pancreatic Pain. Semin Laparosc Surg 1996;3(1):29-33.
4. Davis BR, Vitale M, Lecompte M, Vitale D, Vitale GC. An objective study of pain relief in chronic pancreatitis from bilateral thoracoscopic splanchnicectomy. Am Surg 2008;74(6):510-4.
5. Buscher HC, Schipper EE, Wilder-Smith OH, Jansen JB, van GH. Limited effect of thoracoscopic splanchnicectomy in the treatment of severe chronic pancreatitis pain: a prospective long-term analysis of 75 cases. Surgery 2008; 143(6):715-22.
6. Baghdadi S, Abbas MH, Albouz F, Ammori BJ. Systematic review of the role of thoracoscopic splanchnicectomy in palliating the pain of patients with chronic pancreatitis. Surg Endosc 2008;22(3):580-8.
7. Karanjia ND, Widdison AL, Leung F, Alvarez C, Lutrin FJ, Reber HA. Compartment syndrome in experimental chronic obstructive pancreatitis: effect of decompressing the main pancreatic duct. Br J Surg 1994;81(2):259-64.
8. Yekebas EF, Bogoevski D, Honarpisheh H, Cataldegirmen G, Habermann CR, Seewald S, et al. Long-term follow-up in small duct chronic pancreatitis: A plea for extended drainage by "V-shaped excision" of the anterior aspect of the pancreas. Ann Surg 2006;244(6):940-6.
9. Frey CF, Smith GJ. Description and rationale of a new operation for chronic pancreatitis. Pancreas 1987;2(6):701-7.

10. Beger HG, Krautzberger W, Bittner R, Buchler M, Limmer J. Duodenum-preserving resection of the head of the pancreas in patients with severe chronic pancreatitis. Surgery 1985;97(4):467-73.

11. Warshaw AL. Conservation of the spleen with distal pancreatectomy. Arch Surg 1988;123(5):550-3.

12. Nealon WH, Thompson JC. Progressive loss of pancreatic function in chronic pancreatitis is delayed by main pancreatic duct decompression: A longitudinal prospective analysis of the modified puestow procedure. Ann Surg 1993; 217(5):458-66.

13. Dumonceau JM, Costamagna G, Tringali A, Vahedi K, Delhaye M, Hittelet A, et al. Treatment for painful calcified chronic pancreatitis: extracorporeal shock wave lithotripsy versus endoscopic treatment: a randomised controlled trial. Gut 2007;56(4):545-52.

14. Dite P, Ruzicka M, Zboril V, Novotny I. A prospective, randomized trial comparing endoscopic and surgical therapy for chronic pancreatitis. Endoscopy 2003;35(7):553-8.

15. Cahen DL, Gouma DJ, Nio Y, Rauws EA, Boermeester MA, Busch OR, et al. Endoscopic versus surgical drainage of the pancreatic duct in chronic pancreatitis. N Engl J Med 2007;356(7):676-84.

16. Shah NS, Siriwardena AK. Variance in elective surgery for chronic pancreatitis. JOP 2009;10(1):30-6.

17. Evans JD, Wilson PG, Carver C, Bramhall SR, Buckels JA, Mayer AD, et al. Outcome of surgery for chronic pancreatitis. Br J Surg 1997;84(5):624-9.

18. Keck T, Wellner UF, Riediger H, Adam U, Sick O, Hopt UT, et al. Long-term Outcome after 92 Duodenum-Preserving Pancreatic Head Resections for Chronic Pancreatitis: Comparison of Beger and Frey Procedures. J Gastrointest Surg 2009.

19. Buchler MW, Friess H, Muller MW, Wheatley AM, Beger HG. Randomized trial of duodenum-preserving pancreatic head resection versus pylorus-preserving Whipple in chronic pancreatitis. Am J Surg 1995;169(1):65-9.

20. Farkas G, Leindler L, Daroczi M, Farkas G, Jr. Long-term follow-up after organ-preserving pancreatic head resection in patients with chronic pancreatitis. J Gastrointest Surg 2008;12(2):308-12.

21. Izbicki JR, Bloechle C, Broering DC, Knoefel WT, Kuechler T, Broelsch CE. Extended drainage versus resection in surgery for chronic pancreatitis: a prospective randomized trial comparing the longitudinal pancreaticojejunostomy combined with local pancreatic head excision with the pylorus-preserving pancreatoduodenectomy. Ann Surg 1998;228(6):771-9.

22. Muller MW, Friess H, Martin DJ, Hinz U, Dahmen R, Buchler MW. Long-term follow-up of a randomized clinical trial comparing Beger with pylorus-preserving Whipple procedure for chronic pancreatitis. Br J Surg 2008; 95(3):350-6.

23. Strate T, Taherpour Z, Bloechle C, Mann O, Bruhn JP, Schneider C, et al. Long-term follow-up of a randomized trial comparing the Beger and Frey procedures for patients suffering from chronic pancreatitis. Ann Surg 2005; 241(4):591-8.

24. Strate T, Bachmann K, Busch P, Mann O, Schneider C, Bruhn JP, et al. Resection vs drainage in treatment of chronic pancreatitis: long-term results of a randomized trial. Gastroenterology 2008;134(5):1406-11.

CHAPTER SEVEN

Non-variceal Upper Gastrointestinal Hemorrhage: Advances in Diagnosis and Treatment

Samir P Mehta, James P Byrne

INTRODUCTION

Acute upper gastrointestinal hemorrhage (UGIH), defined as bleeding proximal to the ligament of Treitz, remains a common hospital emergency in the UK, managed primarily by gastroenterologists with surgical input required where appropriate. This review aims to summarize the latest evidence in the management of non-variceal UGIH whilst also outlining improvements in diagnosis and management that have occurred in the last decade. Despite these advances in pharmaceutical and endoscopic treatment there has been little improvement in associated mortality rates.[1] Recently however, there has been excitement over the role of CT angiography in diagnosis and transcatheter embolization as a safe treatment alternative to surgery. These newer modalities are highlighted here and to conclude we propose a novel algorithm for the management of acute UGIH.

Key Point

- Non-variceal hemorrhage remains a common and life threatening clinical condition.

EPIDEMIOLOGY

The crude incidence rates of acute UGIH demonstrate considerable variation across Europe. The highest rates have been recorded in the West of Scotland, 172 per 100,000,[2] and the lowest rates in Demnark[3] and the Netherlands.[4] The incidence is significantly higher in men and rises sharply with age, almost six times higher in those over 75.[5] There are large differences in reported mortality rates across studies. However, there is a broad agreement over the predominant risk factors for mortality which are age, severe comorbidity, presence of shock at initial presentation and re-bleeding.

ETIOLOGY

Peptic ulcer bleeding is the main cause of UGIH and duodenal ulcers are more common than gastric ulcers. The risk factors associated with peptic ulcer disease are primarily *H.pylori* infection and non steroidal anti-inflammatory drug (NSAID) usage. Both of these independently increase the risk of peptic ulcer disease and bleeding, and when both coexist the magnitude of the risk is additive.[6] Over half of UGIH is associated with NSAIDs, but there is no clear link between dosage and incidence.[7] Worryingly, only a small proportion of patients admitted with peptic ulcer bleeding on NSAIDs are also on a proton pump inhibitor (PPI).[8]

Key Point

• Over half of acute UGIH is associated with NSAID usage.

The other less frequent causes of UGIH are listed in Table 7.1. Iatrogenic causes are becoming increasingly important as the number of endoscopic/percutaneous procedures increases particularly in the elderly. With regard to the vascular malformations that can cause UGIH, Dieulafoy's lesions deserve special mention. These are bleeding submucosal vessels with no obvious ulceration. Their importance lies in the fact that they are often difficult to recognize at initial endoscopy and account for a significant percentage of "missed" lesions identified at re-endoscopy.[9]

CLINICAL PRESENTATION AND INITIAL MANAGEMENT

The most common signs are those of melena and hematemesis, although the presence of this does not always exclude hemorrhage from a site distal to the ligament of Treitz. Other symptoms depend on the cause. For example, epigastric pain may be associated with peptic ulcer disease,

TABLE 7.1

Main causes of upper gastrointestinal bleeding

Cause	Frequency (%)
Duodenal ulcer	25
Gastric ulcer	15
Erosions	15
Varices	15
Esophagitis / gastritis	7
Mallory Weiss tear	6
Vascular malformations	5
Upper GI malignancy	3
Other (including iatrogenic)	9

preceding weight loss and dysphagia with upper gastrointestinal malignancy. A recent history of vomiting or retching might be suggestive of a Mallory-Weiss tear.

Initial clinical assessment should focus on the hemodynamic status of the patient and must include assessment of pulse rate, blood pressure and capillary refill time. Treatment should be aimed at volume replacement and airway protection, the latter being particularly important in those with significant hematemesis. Blood transfusion should be instituted appropriately according to hemodynamic parameters. When indicated the correction of coagulopathy is also important. Hemoglobin levels may be misleading in the acute situation and correlate poorly with the risk of rebleeding or subsequent mortality. Hematocrit may be useful as a measure of dilution. There is a growing body of evidence that a less vigorous approach to transfusion in UGIH may actually be beneficial, in promoting hemostasis.[10] However, given the conventional recommendation of liberal volume, resuscitation in UGIH, it has been difficult to evaluate the role of a restricted transfusion.

Frequently, there is diagnostic uncertainty during the initial assessment. Insertion of a wide bore nasogastric tube and examination of the aspirate may yield important predictive information regarding the location of bleeding and in particular whether the patient requires urgent endoscopic evaluation.[11] The decision of when to perform endoscopy is essentially based on clinical judgement and should be discussed with the duty endoscopist.

PATIENT STRATIFICATION

There have been a number of scoring systems that have been developed to identify patients that are at high risk of either requiring specific treatments, or of rebleeding or death. Such scores are no doubt useful as adjuncts to clinical evaluation and judgement and can also be particularly useful in identifying patients who are at low risk of complications and who may be suitable for early discharge.[12] These scores range from those based on simple endoscopic criteria, such as that by Forrest et al[13] (Table 7.2), to pre-endoscopic clinical scores, such as the Blatchford[14] score through to combine clinical and endoscopic evaluation, such as the Rockall scoring system.[15]

The combined Rockall score (Table 7.3) was published in 1996 and is probably the most widely known scoring system. It has been revalidated across a number of units worldwide but there have been discrepancies with regard to the score being able to predict mortality and risk of rebleeding; this is especially true at higher scores.[16,17] The score consists of an initial calculation based on age, presence of comorbidity and presence of shock with additional stratification based on the bleeding lesion and endoscopic stigmata of hemorrhage. A total score of less than

TABLE 7.2

Modified Forrest classification for upper GI hemorrhage

Class	Endoscopic findings	Re-bleed rate (%)	Endoscopic treatment recommended
Ia	Spurting artery	80-90	Yes
Ib	Oozing hemorrhage	10-30	Yes
IIa	Non-bleeding visible vessel	50-60	Yes
IIb	Adherent clot	25-35	Debatable
IIc	Ulcer base with black spot sign	0-8	No
III	Clean base	0-12	No

TABLE 7.3

Rockall scoring system for upper GI hemorrhage

	Score			
Variable	0	1	2	3
Age/yrs	<60	60-79	>79	
Shock	No shock	Tachycardia (pulse > 100)	Tachycardia (pulse > 100) Hypotension (systolic < 100)	
Comorbidity	None		Ischemic heart disease Cardiac failure	Renal failure Liver failure Disseminated malignancy
Diagnosis	Mallory Weiss No lesion No stigmata of recent	All other diagnoses except malignancy hemorrhage	Upper GI malignancy	
Endoscopic findings	None Dark spot sign		Blood in upper GI tract Adherent clot Visible/spurting vessel	

A score of 3 or less = low risk; score of >8 = high risk

3 is associated with an excellent outcome whereas a score of higher than 8 is associated with a high mortality (Table 7.3).

MEDICAL TREATMENT

Proton pump inhibition (PPI) has been shown to improve outcome in peptic ulcer bleeding and there is some evidence to support commencement of PPI treatment prior to endoscopy.[18] A recent Cochrane review has shown that patients, receiving PPI treatment are less likely to have endoscopic evidence of high-risk stigmata compared to placebo.[19] The underlying basis for using such drugs comes from *in vitro* studies, demonstrating that platelet aggregation was inhibited by acid and that increasing the intragastric pH could improve the coagulation process.[20] *In vivo* studies have demonstrated that an infusion of omeprazole can maintain a pH of above 6 during the initial 72 hours period.[21] The recommended dose is 80 mg bolus of omeprazole followed by an infusion of 8mg/h intravenously over 72 hours.[22] Subsequently, Lau et al have shown that following hemostasis achieved at endoscopy, high dose omeprazole infusion reduced the rate of rebleeding and duration of hospitalization.[23] Recent meta-analyses have confirmed Lau's results, but there is no clear evidence that PPI treatment alone decreases overall mortality,[24,25] and the reduction of mortality in certain studies appears to be only among patients with high-risk stigmata who have initially undergone endoscopic therapy.[26]

Key Points

- High dose PPI infusion reduces the risk of rebleeding and length of hospital stay.
- Octreotide may reduce the risk of rebleeding and need for surgery. Tranexamic acid may have a role in the management of acute UGIH although this has not yet been proven.

A recent meta-analysis has found that histamine receptor antagonists are of no benefit in preventing risk of rebleeding or in reducing mortality.[27] This may be explained by the fact that although these drugs are effective in increasing intragastric pH above 6 at least initially, continuous intravenous infusion results in gastric tolerance within the first 12 hours.[28] Somatostatin analogs, such as octreotide may have a role in the management of acute UGIH. A recent meta-analysis randomized controlled trials (RCT) covering 14 has shown some evidence for octreotide reducing the risk of continued bleeding and a trend towards reducing the need for surgery.[29]

Tranexamic acid is an antifibrinolytic agent that inhibits plasminogen activators. A recent systematic review looking at 7 RCTs has reported that tranexamic acid may reduce mortality, but there were limitations in the validity of the included trials.[30] Thus, tranexamic acid cannot currently be recommended in the medical management of UGIH.

ENDOSCOPIC MANAGEMENT

Early endoscopy for low-risk patients may be beneficial in facilitating prompt discharge.[31] For high-risk patients there is some evidence that early endoscopy (i.e. within 12 hours) may reduce rebleeding and surgery rates.[32,33] In cases of severe bleeding erythromycin administration up to an hour before endoscopy may improve the evaluation of the upper gastrointestinal tract through its prokinetic properties.[34] Caution is required in selecting patients for endoscopy within 12 hours of admission because of the increased risk of aspiration of gastric contents during endoscopy.

Key Point

- Endoscopy is the first line intervention and the majority of patients will not require any further treatment.

The goal of early endoscopy is to determine the cause of bleeding, identify prognostic features and in those that have high risk stigmata (active bleeding or a visible vessel) administer therapy, since there is a high risk of rebleeding without treatment.[35] There is some debate with regard to whether an adherent clot should be treated. A recent prospective study showed no benefit from endoscopic treatment of these lesions in individuals treated with high dose PPI.[26] Ulcers with a black spot or clean base are associated with a low risk of rebleeding and do not require endoscopic therapy.

Key Point

- Early endoscopy facilitates prompt discharge in low-risk patients and reduces the risk of rebleeding in high-risk patients.

TECHNIQUES FOR ENDOSCOPIC THERAPY

In general, no single endoscopic therapy has been identified to be superior to any of the others, but all have been shown to be superior to no intervention.[22,36] For high-risk lesions however a combination of adrenaline injection plus thermal treatment has been shown to be superior to monotherapy in RCTs.[37,38] Indeed, the prior injection of adrenaline may arrest the rate of bleeding, thus, allowing better visibility for targeted thermal therapy.

Mechanical devices, in particular endoscopic clips used in conjunction with adrenaline, have been shown to be superior to injection therapy alone in a recent randomized trial.[39] However, endoscopic clips can be difficult to apply and can be technically demanding depending on the nature of the ulcer itself. Clip placement during endoscopy however may help to localize the culprit vessel if angiography is planned subsequently.[40] The exact roles of newer and emerging techniques, such as endoscopic suturing, stapling devices and cryotherapy remain to be clarified in appropriately powered studies.

Recently a variety of gastroscopes have become available either with a single large caliber channel or with dual channels. Their primary advantage is in allowing effective suction. Occasionally, the side viewing duodenoscope may be useful in visualizing lesions particularly at the D1/D2 interface.

Therapeutic endoscopy can achieve hemostasis in over 70% of cases.[41] A planned second look endoscopy, performed within 24 hours, does not alter either the risk of mortality or need for surgery,[42] although many clinicians would schedule a second look in certain high-risk patients. A re-look is also useful in predicting further recurrent bleeding, if endoscopic factors, such as large ulcer size and stigmata of recent hemorrhage persist at the time of the second endoscopy.[43]

MULTIDETECTOR ROW CT (MDCT) SCANNING

Traditionally, endoscopy has been considered to be the main diagnostic tool in acute gastrointestinal hemorrhage. However, in a proportion of patients it is impossible to make the diagnosis through endoscopy either because of excessive bleeding or clots or because the bleeding may be coming from further distally in the GI tract. Recent technological improvements in CT scanning (thinner collimation, faster scanning times for instance) have highlighted the growing role of MDCT scanning in patients with acute GI hemorrhage. A recent prospective study from Italy has demonstrated improved sensitivity in identifying etiology of bleeding by MDCT as compared with endoscopy in upper gastrointestinal hemorrhage.[44] MDCT is particularly sensitive in identifying bleeding from the small bowel. These authors have proposed an algorithm in which MDCT should be the initial investigation in patients with acute gastrointestinal bleeding rather than endoscopy. Further prospective studies to validate these results are eagerly awaited.

Key Point

- Multi-detector CT has high sensitivity in identifying the source of bleeding throughout the gastrointestinal tract.

PERSISTENT AND RECURRENT BLEEDING

Failure to achieve primary hemostasis because of torrential bleeding or if visibility is obscured for any other reason has conventionally been an indication for immediate surgery. This is certainly true for massive hemorrhage precluding stabilization prior to endoscopy. In this situation, endoscopy should be performed in the operating theater. Although surgery can be a gratifying means of controlling hemorrhage, it is associated with a mortality rate approaching 30%.[45]

Selective angioembolization has been proposed as an alternative to surgery and is currently considered as a first line treatment for colonic bleeding,[46] the obvious advantage being the avoidance of a laparotomy particularly in the critically ill patient. The techniques available are described below.

ANGIOGRAPHY WITH TRANSCATHETER EMBOLIZATION

In the UGIT angiography with transcatheter embolization was first described in 1972.[47] Since then it has been used predominantly in situations where endoscopy has failed to control bleeding and surgery is not appropriate.[48] Embolization is particularly useful in patients that are too sick to undergo surgery. Indeed in patients with multiorgan failure successful embolization offers the only chance of survival.[49]

Recently however, there have been a number of published reports of case series where the technique has been utilized as an effective means of controlling hemorrhage in patients where the location of bleeding is unknown but also in those where bleeding cannot be controlled at endoscopy. The most recent of these (within the last 10 years) are listed in Table 7.4. Many of these studies have reported success in the absence of contrast extravasation (so called "blind" embolization) although this is a controversial area. Holme et al[50] reported a 61% clinical success rate of embolization of the gastroduodenal artery in patients with negative angiograms. Others have recommended embolization of the left gastric artery if bleeding is thought to emanate from this vascular territory.[51]

The risk of significant ischemia following embolization is low because of the rich collateral blood supply to the stomach and duodenum. However, this risk is increased in patients who have had a history of surgery in the area,[52] or with embolic agents that can advance far into the vascular bed, such as tissue adhesives and gelatin powder. The combination of coils and embolic particles has recently been more widely used because of their reduced distal occlusive properties.

Although there have never been any randomized comparisons, in a recent retrospective study from Sweden there was a clear trend towards a lower 30 day mortality in patients that were embolized compared to those having surgery following failed endoscopic treatment.[53] One of the major risk factors for mortality following transcatheter embolization is early rebleeding.[54] Furthermore, coagulopathy also correlates with failure and death, supporting the notion that thrombus formation is essential for success.[49,55] Finally, the need for rescue surgery following failed embolization also appears to be a risk factor for mortality.[55]

TABLE 7.4

Published series of angiographic embolization for upper gastrointestinal hemorrhage

Source	Year	No. of patients	Technical success rate	Re-bleed rate	Mortality	comments
Padia et al[56]	2009	108	100%	56%	22%	Arterial embolization was equally effective in patients who demonstrate contrast extravasation during angiography compared to those who do not
Loffroy et al[57]	2009	60	95%	28%	27%	Retrospective series. Extravasation of contrast in 38 patients. No extravasation in 22 patients. Coagulation disorders and use of coils alone were independent predictors of embolization failure
Poultsides et al[58]	2008	57	94%	49%	21%	Retrospective review of patients referred after endoscopic treatment failure. Angiographic failure was more likely if embolization was performed late, following massive blood transfusion and for re-hemorrhage after suture ligation of duodenal ulcer
Holme et al[50]	2006	40	100%	35%	25%	Referrals for embolotherapy after unsuccessful endoscopic or surgical treatment. 70% did not have extravasation on angiography but were embolized anyway
Ripoll et al[59]	2004	31	100%	29%	26%	Retrospective comparison of embolotherapy versus surgery after therapeutic endoscopy failure. No difference in outcome between groups
Ljungdahl et al[60]	2002	18 (13 after endo-scopic failure, 5 after surgery)	100%	17%	6%	Prospective case series. 5 patients had no evidence of contrast extravasation but were embolized (either GDA or LGA)

Contd...

Table contd...

Source	Year	No. of patients	Technical success rate	Re-bleed rate	Mortality	Comments
Aina et al[55]	2001	75	99%	24%	35%	Case series. Bleeding detected at endoscopy and angiography in 22 patients, endoscopy alone in 29 patients and angiography alone in 24 patients.Coagulopathy and the use of coils alone were associated with higher risk of recurrent bleeding
Defreyne et al[61]	2001	40	98%	32%	28%	Retrospective analysis of 40 patients who underwent arteriography following endoscopically unmanageable non-variceal UGIH
Schenker et al[49]	2001	163	95%	42%	33%	Retrospective review of all patients over a 12 yr period. Multiorgan failure, coagulopathy and bleeding subsequent to trauma / invasive procedure were negatively associated with survival
Walsh et al[62]	2001	50	92%	48%	40%	Retrospective review of patients who underwent angiography in UGIH not controlled at endoscopy. Patients who had a shorter time to angiography had better survival outcome

Note: GDA gastroduodenal artery, LGA left gastric artery

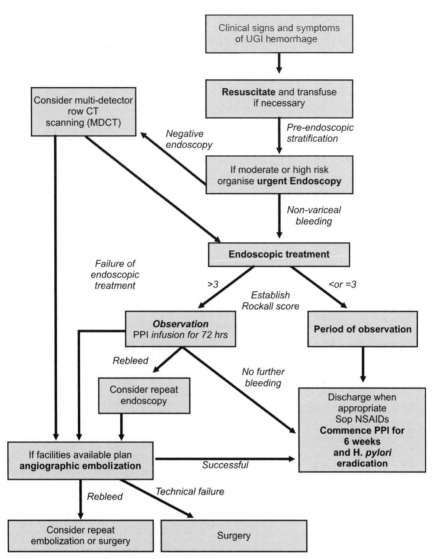

Fig. 7.1: Proposed algorithm for the management of non-variceal upper GI hemorrhage.

Key Points

- Transcatheter embolization may offer advantages, compared to surgery following failed endoscopic therapy.
- Transcatheter embolization is best provided in high volume centers where there are experienced interventional radiologists.
- A proportion of patients will always require definitive surgical management.

Most of the studies listed in Table 7.4 have included small numbers of patients and have not separated peptic ulcer bleeding from other causes. Furthermore, there is no consensus in the literature on the ideal choice of embolic agent. The low postoperative morbidity is one of the main advantages of transcatheter embolization over surgery. However, there will always be some patients who ultimately require a definitive surgical procedure.

In high volume centers where there are experienced interventional radiologists available, it is now clear that angiographic embolization can be used as a nonoperative adjunct in order to avoid surgery. The available evidence would certainly support the algorithm illustrated in Figure 7.1, although as yet there have been no randomized trials comparing angiographic transcatheter embolization with surgery following failed endoscopic therapy.

REFERENCES

1. Vreeburg EM, Snel P, de Bruijne JW, Bartelsman JF, Rauws EA, Tytgat GN. Acute upper gastrointestinal bleeding in the Amsterdam area: incidence, diagnosis, and clinical outcome. Am J Gastroenterol 1997;92(2):236-43.
2. Blatchford O, Davidson LA, Murray WR, Blatchford M, Pell J. Acute upper gastrointestinal hemorrhage in west of Scotland: case ascertainment study. Bmj 1997;315(7107):510-4.
3. Nielsen GL, Sorensen HT, Mellemkjoer L, Blot WJ, McLaughlin JK, Tage-Jensen U, et al. Risk of hospitalization resulting from upper gastrointestinal bleeding among patients taking corticosteroids: a register-based cohort study. Am J Med 2001;111(7):541-5.
4. van Leerdam ME. Epidemiology of acute upper gastrointestinal bleeding. Best Pract Res Clin Gastroenterol 2008;22(2):209-24.
5. Longstreth GF. Epidemiology of hospitalization for acute gastro-intestinal hemorrhage: a population-based study. Am J Gastroenterol 1995; 90(2):206-10.
6. Huang JQ, Sridhar S, Hunt RH. Role of Helicobacter pylori infection and non-steroidal anti-inflammatory drugs in peptic-ulcer disease: a meta-analysis. Lancet 2002;359(9300):14-22.
7. Rollhauser C, Fleischer DE. Nonvariceal upper gastrointestinal bleeding. Endoscopy 2002;34(2):111-8.
8. Ramsoekh D, van Leerdam ME, Rauws EA, Tytgat GN. Outcome of peptic ulcer bleeding, nonsteroidal anti-inflammatory drug use, and Helicobacter pylori infection. Clin Gastroenterol Hepatol 2005;3(9):859-64.
9. Chung YF, Wong WK, Soo KC. Diagnostic failures in endoscopy for acute upper gastrointestinal hemorrhage. Br J Surg 2000;87(5):614-7.
10. Duggan JM. Gastrointestinal hemorrhage: should we transfuse less? Dig Dis Sci 2009;54(8):1662-6.
11. Aljebreen AM, Fallone CA, Barkun AN. Nasogastric aspirate predicts high-risk endoscopic lesions in patients with acute upper-GI bleeding. Gastrointest Endosc 2004;59(2):172-8.

12. Atkinson RJ, Hurlstone DP. Usefulness of prognostic indices in upper gastro-intestinal bleeding. Best Pract Res Clin Gastroenterol 2008;22(2):233-42.

13. Forrest JA, Finlayson ND, Shearman DJ. Endoscopy in gastrointestinal bleeding. Lancet 1974;2(7877):394-7.

14. Blatchford O, Murray WR, Blatchford M. A risk score to predict need for treatment for upper-gastrointestinal hemorrhage. Lancet 2000;356(9238):1318-21.

15. Rockall TA, Logan RF, Devlin HB, Northfield TC. Risk assessment after acute upper gastrointestinal hemorrhage. Gut 1996;38(3):316-21.

16. Enns RA, Gagnon YM, Barkun AN, Armstrong D, Gregor JC, Fedorak RN. Validation of the Rockall scoring system for outcomes from non-variceal upper gastrointestinal bleeding in a Canadian setting. World J Gastroenterol 2006;12(48):7779-85.

17. Sarwar S, Dilshad A, Khan AA, Alam A, Butt AK, Tariq S, et al. Predictive value of Rockall score for rebleeding and mortality in patients with variceal bleeding. J Coll Physicians Surg Pak 2007;17(5):253-6.

18. Andrews CN, Levy A, Fishman M, Hahn M, Atkinson K, Kwan P, et al. Intravenous proton pump inhibitors before endoscopy in bleeding peptic ulcer with high-risk stigmata: a multicentre comparative study. Can J Gastro-enterol 2005;19(11):667-71.

19. Dorward S, Sreedharan A, Leontiadis GI, Howden CW, Moayyedi P, Forman D. Proton pump inhibitor treatment initiated prior to endoscopic diagnosis in upper gastrointestinal bleeding. Cochrane Database Syst Rev 2006(4):CD005415.

20. Green FW, Jr., Kaplan MM, Curtis LE, Levine PH. Effect of acid and pepsin on blood coagulation and platelet aggregation. A possible contributor prolonged gastroduodenal mucosal hemorrhage. Gastroenterology 1978;74(1):38-43.

21. Netzer P, Gaia C, Sandoz M, Huluk T, Gut A, Halter F, et al. Effect of repeated injection and continuous infusion of omeprazole and ranitidine on intragastric pH over 72 hours. Am J Gastroenterol 1999;94(2):351-7.

22. Barkun A, Bardou M, Marshall JK. Consensus recommendations for managing patients with nonvariceal upper gastrointestinal bleeding. Ann Intern Med 2003;139(10):843-57.

23. Lau JY, Sung JJ, Lee KK, Yung MY, Wong SK, Wu JC, et al. Effect of intravenous omeprazole on recurrent bleeding after endoscopic treatment of bleeding peptic ulcers. N Engl J Med 2000;343(5):310-6.

24. Leontiadis GI, Sharma VK, Howden CW. Systematic review and meta-analysis of proton pump inhibitor therapy in peptic ulcer bleeding. BMJ 2005;330(7491):568.

25. Andriulli A, Annese V, Caruso N, Pilotto A, Accadia L, Niro AG, et al. Proton-pump inhibitors and outcome of endoscopic hemostasis in bleeding peptic ulcers: a series of meta-analyses. Am J Gastroenterol 2005;100(1):207-19.

26. Sung JJ, Chan FK, Lau JY, Yung MY, Leung WK, Wu JC, et al. The effect of endoscopic therapy in patients receiving omeprazole for bleeding ulcers with nonbleeding visible vessels or adherent clots: a randomized comparison. Ann Intern Med 2003;139(4):237-43.

27. Levine JE, Leontiadis GI, Sharma VK, Howden CW. Meta-analysis: the efficacy of intravenous H2-receptor antagonists in bleeding peptic ulcer. Aliment Pharmacol Ther 2002;16(6):1137-42.

28. Labenz J, Peitz U, Leusing C, Tillenburg B, Blum AL, Borsch G. Efficacy of primed infusions with high dose ranitidine and omeprazole to maintain high intragastric pH in patients with peptic ulcer bleeding: a prospective randomised controlled study. Gut 1997;40(1):36-41.

29. May G, Butler J. The Use of vasoconstrictor therapy in non-variceal upper GI bleeds. Emerg Med J 2006;23(9):722-4.

30. Gluud LL, Klingenberg SL, Langholz SE. Systematic review: tranexamic acid for upper gastrointestinal bleeding. Aliment Pharmacol Ther 2008; 27(9):752-8.

31. Cipolletta L, Bianco MA, Rotondano G, Marmo R, Piscopo R. Outpatient management for low-risk nonvariceal upper GI bleeding: a randomized controlled trial. Gastrointest Endosc 2002;55(1):1-5.

32. Cooper GS, Chak A, Connors AF, Jr., Harper DL, Rosenthal GE. The effectiveness of early endoscopy for upper gastrointestinal hemorrhage: a community-based analysis. Med Care 1998;36(4):462-74.

33. Cooper GS, Chak A, Way LE, Hammar PJ, Harper DL, Rosenthal GE. Early endoscopy in upper gastrointestinal hemorrhage: associations with recurrent bleeding, surgery, and length of hospital stay. Gastrointest Endosc 1999;49(2):145-52.

34. Frossard JL, Spahr L, Queneau PE, Giostra E, Burckhardt B, Ory G, et al. Erythromycin intravenous bolus infusion in acute upper gastrointestinal bleeding: a randomized, controlled, double-blind trial. Gastroenterology 2002;123(1):17-23.

35. Laine L, Peterson WL. Bleeding peptic ulcer. N Engl J Med 1994;331(11):717-27.

36. Adler DG, Leighton JA, Davila RE, Hirota WK, Jacobson BC, Qureshi WA, et al. ASGE guideline: The role of endoscopy in acute non-variceal upper-GI hemorrhage. Gastrointest Endosc 2004;60(4):497-504.

37. Calvet X, Vergara M, Brullet E, Gisbert JP, Campo R. Addition of a second endoscopic treatment following epinephrine injection improves outcome in high-risk bleeding ulcers. Gastroenterology 2004;126(2):441-50.

38. Lin HJ, Tseng GY, Perng CL, Lee FY, Chang FY, Lee SD. Comparison of adrenaline injection and bipolar electrocoagulation for the arrest of peptic ulcer bleeding. Gut 1999;44(5):715-9.

39. Park CH, Joo YE, Kim HS, Choi SK, Rew JS, Kim SJ. A prospective, randomized trial comparing mechanical methods of hemostasis plus epinephrine injection to epinephrine injection alone for bleeding peptic ulcer. Gastrointest Endosc 2004;60(2):173-9.

40. Eriksson LG, Sundbom M, Gustavsson S, Nyman R. Endoscopic marking with a metallic clip facilitates transcatheter arterial embolization in upper peptic ulcer bleeding. J Vasc Interv Radiol 2006;17(6):959-64.

41. Ferguson CB, Mitchell RM. Nonvariceal upper gastrointestinal bleeding: standard and new treatment. Gastroenterol Clin North Am 2005;34(4):607-21.

42. Marmo R, Rotondano G, Bianco MA, Piscopo R, Prisco A, Cipolletta L. Outcome of endoscopic treatment for peptic ulcer bleeding: Is a second look necessary? A meta-analysis. Gastrointest Endosc 2003;57(1):62-7.

43. Chiu PW, Joeng HK, Choi CL, Kwong KH, Ng EK, Lam SH. Predictors of peptic ulcer rebleeding after scheduled second endoscopy: clinical or endoscopic factors? Endoscopy 2006;38(7):726-9.

44. Frattaroli FM, Casciani E, Spoletini D, Polettini E, Nunziale A, Bertini L, et al. Prospective study comparing multi-detector row CT and endoscopy in acute gastrointestinal bleeding. World J Surg 2009;33(10):2209-17.

45. Poxon VA, Keighley MR, Dykes PW, Heppinstall K, Jaderberg M. Comparison of minimal and conventional surgery in patients with bleeding peptic ulcer: a multicentre trial. Br J Surg 1991;78(11):1344-5.

46. DeBarros J, Rosas L, Cohen J, Vignati P, Sardella W, Hallisey M. The changing paradigm for the treatment of colonic hemorrhage: superselective angiographic embolization. Dis Colon Rectum 2002;45(6):802-8.

47. Rosch J, Dotter CT, Brown MJ. Selective arterial embolization. A new method for control of acute gastrointestinal bleeding. Radiology 1972;102(2):303-6.

48. Lieberman DA, Keller FS, Katon RM, Rosch J. Arterial embolization for massive upper gastrointestinal tract bleeding in poor surgical candidates. Gastroenterology 1984;86(5 Pt 1):876-85.

49. Schenker MP, Duszak R, Jr., Soulen MC, Smith KP, Baum RA, Cope C, et al. Upper gastrointestinal hemorrhage and transcatheter embolotherapy: clinical and technical factors impacting success and survival. J Vasc Interv Radiol 2001;12(11):1263-71.

50. Holme JB, Nielsen DT, Funch-Jensen P, Mortensen FV. Transcatheter arterial embolization in patients with bleeding duodenal ulcer: an alternative to surgery. Acta Radiol 2006;47(3):244-7.

51. Lang EV, Picus D, Marx MV, Hicks ME, Friedland GW. Massive upper gastrointestinal hemorrhage with normal findings on arteriography: value of prophylactic embolization of the left gastric artery. AJR Am J Roentgenol 1992;158(3):547-9.

52. Shapiro N, Brandt L, Sprayregan S, Mitsudo S, Glotzer P. Duodenal infarction after therapeutic Gelfoam embolization of a bleeding duodenal ulcer. Gastroenterology 1981;80(1):176-80.

53. Eriksson LG, Ljungdahl M, Sundbom M, Nyman R. Transcatheter arterial embolization versus surgery in the treatment of upper gastrointestinal bleeding after therapeutic endoscopy failure. J Vasc Interv Radiol 2008;19(10):1413-8.

54. Dempsey DT, Burke DR, Reilly RS, McLean GK, Rosato EF. Angiography in poor-risk patients with massive nonvariceal upper gastrointestinal bleeding. Am J Surg 1990;159(3):282-6.

55. Aina R, Oliva VL, Therasse E, Perreault P, Bui BT, Dufresne MP, et al. Arterial embolotherapy for upper gastrointestinal hemorrhage: outcome assessment. J Vasc Interv Radiol 2001;12(2):195-200.

56. Padia SA, Geisinger MA, Newman JS, Pierce G, Obuchowski NA, Sands MJ. Effectiveness of coil embolization in angiographically detectable versus non-detectable sources of upper gastrointestinal hemorrhage. J Vasc Interv Radiol 2009;20(4):461-6.

57. Loffroy R, Guiu B, D'Athis P, Mezzetta L, Gagnaire A, Jouve JL, et al. Arterial embolotherapy for endoscopically unmanageable acute gastroduodenal hemorrhage: predictors of early rebleeding. Clin Gastroenterol Hepatol 2009;7(5):515-23.

58. Poultsides GA, Kim CJ, Orlando R, 3rd, Peros G, Hallisey MJ, Vignati PV. Angiographic embolization for gastroduodenal hemorrhage: safety, efficacy, and predictors of outcome. Arch Surg 2008;143(5):457-61.

59. Ripoll C, Banares R, Beceiro I, Menchen P, Catalina MV, Echenagusia A, et al. Comparison of transcatheter arterial embolization and surgery for treatment of bleeding peptic ulcer after endoscopic treatment failure. J Vasc Interv Radiol 2004;15(5):447-50.

60. Ljungdahl M, Eriksson LG, Nyman R, Gustavsson S. Arterial embolisation in management of massive bleeding from gastric and duodenal ulcers. Eur J Surg 2002;168(7):384-90.

61. Defreyne L, Vanlangenhove P, De Vos M, Pattyn P, Van Maele G, Decruyenaere J, et al. Embolization as a first approach with endoscopically unmanageable acute nonvariceal gastrointestinal hemorrhage. Radiology 2001;218(3):739-48.

62. Walsh RM, Anain P, Geisinger M, Vogt D, Mayes J, Grundfest-Broniatowski S, et al. Role of angiography and embolization for massive gastroduodenal hemorrhage. J Gastrointest Surg 1999;3(1):61-5; discussion 66.

SECTION FIVE

COLORECTAL

CHAPTER EIGHT

Colonic Pseudo-obstruction

Peter J Lunniss, Charles H Knowles

INTRODUCTION

Colonic pseudo-obstruction refers to the massive dilatation of the colon with obstructive symptoms but in the absence of a mechanical cause. This can occur acutely and may be a component of ileus in which the small bowel is also dilated, or chronically, either individually, usually termed megacolon,[1] or as part of a more generalized visceral dilatation termed chronic intestinal pseudo-obstruction.[2] This chapter will focus on acute colonic pseudo-obstruction, specifically addressing recent advances in clinical management.

HISTORICAL CONSIDERATIONS

Although earlier reports exist, description of the clinical syndrome, now referred to as acute colonic pseudo-obstruction, is generally accredited to Ogilvie in 1948 when he recognized the clinical picture associated with retroperitoneal malignancy, speculating that loss of prevertebral ganglionic sympathetic input might be the cause. Hence, the eponym Ogilvie's syndrome.[3] The term 'pseudo-obstruction' itself was adopted in 1958, having been reported in the Journal of the Royal College of Surgeons of Edinburgh.[2] A series of 13 rather heterogeneous patients was described, including some (in current taxonomy) with postoperative ileus, acute colonic pseudo-obstruction, chronic idiopathic intestinal pseudo-obstruction and megacolon. The full descriptive term 'acute colonic pseudo-obstruction' was first used in 1982 by an Italian Group.[4] The use of eponyms in general is now discouraged, however many surgeons generally favor them as *aide memoires*. Thus, while the authors would tend to encourage the alternative term of Ogilvie's syndrome to describe acute pseudo-obstruction, it should be noted that 'purists' might criticize the uninitiated trainees who (mis)use the term to include patients other than those with retroperitoneal neoplasia (very rare).

DEFINITIONS

The diagnosis of acute colonic pseudo-obstruction is not one that should be made glibly. Fundamental to the definition is the exclusion of the numerous patients referred to surgeons from various hospital departments (often psychiatry, care of the elderly) in whom dilatation of the colon arises either as a result of distal fecal loading (a form of subacute mechanical obstruction) or those in whom painless abdominal distension occurs in the absence of mechanical cause, but without the cardinal symptoms and signs of large bowel obstruction. The latter are troublesome to the trainee, first because the patient will often have a pattern of clinical comorbidities, for example senility, neurological disease and drugs affecting gut motility akin to those associated with the development of acute colonic pseudo-obstruction and secondly, because the referring doctor will almost certainly present a plain radiograph showing significant colonic dilatation.

Key Point

- A diagnosis of acute colonic pseudo-obstruction cannot be made on the basis of bowel dilatation alone. The patient must also be clinically obstructed.

EPIDEMIOLOGY

The exact prevalence of acute colonic pseudo-obstruction is unknown, but can be related to the incidence of large bowel obstruction where it is responsible for at least 20% of cases,[5,6] or by its frequency of complicating other operations. It occurs in about 1% of hospitalized patients undergoing orthopedic procedures, including lower limb joint replacement and spinal operation[7] and in 0.3% of patients with severe burns.[8] The highest prevalence is observed in the late middle age (60 years) being slightly more frequent in males (60% of cases). Acute colonic pseudo-obstruction is a severe condition with considerable clinical and social impact. Published data[9] and reviews clearly show that because of multiple comorbidities, delayed diagnosis and inappropriate treatment, it is responsible for high morbidity and mortality (25-31% overall and 40-50% with ischemia or perforation).[9-11]

ETIOLOGY

Most patients develop acute colonic pseudo-obstruction in association with one or more of a wide array of clinical conditions. Large retrospective evaluations[9,12] have demonstrated that operative (23%) and non-operative trauma (11%), infections (10%) and cardiac disease (10% to 18%) were the most common predisposing conditions. In reality, most patients fall into one of two groups; younger patients with spinal and other trauma,

TABLE 8.1

Etiological factors in acute colonic pseudo-obstruction

Typically younger		Typically older	
Postoperative	Spinal surgery	Neurological	Parkinson's disease
	Pelvic/hip surgery		Alzheimer's disease
	Renal transplantation		Multiple sclerosis
	Cesarean section		Stroke
Post-traumatic agents	Spinal cord injury Pelvic and femoral fractures	Neuroactive drugs	Anti-Parkinsonian Opioid analgesics
SIRS/MODS	Mechanical ventilation		Phenothiazines
	Polytrauma		Antidepressants
	Sepsis	Cardiac	Myocardial infarction
	Acute pancreatitis		Cardiac failure

including operative and older patients with multiple chronic comorbidities (Table 8.1). The pathogenesis of acute colonic pseudo-obstruction remains unclear but is generally considered (without much real direct evidence) to relate to an imbalance of extrinsic (autonomic) visceral innervation. The clinical response to neostigmine (below) indirectly points to parasympathetic dysfunction perhaps being more important than sympathetic overactivity. Interestingly, the intrinsic (enteric nervous system) inhibitory motor neurotransmitter nitrous oxide has been shown to be overproduced in patients with toxic megacolon[13] but has not been studied in acute colonic pseudo-obstruction. A fuller synopsis of the neurogastroenterological aspects of this condition has been recently published.[14]

CLINICAL PRESENTATION AND INVESTIGATION

Acute colonic pseudo-obstruction is characterized by significant abdominal distension, pain, nausea and/or vomiting, with failure to pass flatus or stools documented in up to 60% of patients.[9,11,12] Due to the presence of massive colonic dilatation, ischemia and perforation may occur with subsequent clinical findings of peritonism. Such complications occur in 3 to 15% of patients,[9,11,12] advanced age, cecal diameter and delay in decompression increase the risk. Despite the best critical care, the mortality of these complications runs around 50%. Physical examination in uncomplicated cases commonly reveals a tympanic non-tender abdomen with high-pitched 'tinkling', reduced or absent bowel sounds. On digital examination of the rectum, it is usually found to be grossly voluminous and empty—"you can't touch the sides" (in contrast to mechanical obstruction when it is usually collapsed). Patients with complications present with marked abdominal tenderness and systemic features, such

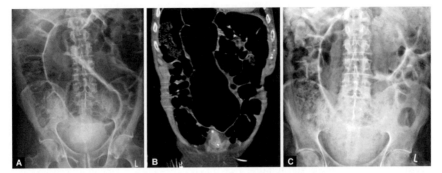

Figs 8.1A to C: (A) Plain abdominal radiograph of 73 year-old male with acute colonic pseudo-obstruction associated with antipsychotic medication and Parkinson's disease, (B) CT scan with rectal catheter and contrast and (C) the same patient after repeat presentation 3 weeks later (pseudo-obstruction had recurred despite successful colonoscopic decompression on the last admission).

as fever and tachycardia. The differential diagnosis in hospitalized or institutionalized patients includes mechanical obstruction and increasingly toxic megacolon due to *Clostridium difficile* infection, which should always be excluded by appropriate stool testing.[15]

Diagnosis relies upon accurate clinical observation and plain abdominal radiography showing degrees of colonic dilatation, mainly involving the proximal colon (Figs 8.1A and C).[16-18] Plain abdominal and chest radiographs can give some indication of colonic diameter, as well as detecting the presence of free air suggestive of perforation. However, in all cases of large bowel obstruction, however clear the diagnosis appears on plain radiology, a water soluble contrast enema (WSCE)[5,6] (Fig. 8.1B) or contrast CT scan[19] (Fig. 8.1B) must be performed in addition to a rigid sigmoidoscopy to differentiate mechanical from pseudo-obstruction and thus prevent injudicious laparotomy for a non-existent cancer. No direct comparison has been made between these imaging modalities in terms of diagnostic accuracy, however both have very high rates of accuracy with respect to differentiating mechanical from pseudo-obstruction as determined ultimately by surgery - WSCE: sensitivity 96% and specificity 98%;[18] CT (with IV contrast only): 91% specificity and sensitivity.[20] CT has the additional advantages of giving more accurate bowel diameter measurements[20,21] and better information on the mucosal condition both in terms of detection of co-existent inflammation and of viability. Ischemic changes may be evident as wall thickening, submucosal edema and with advancing necrosis and intramural gas. Adjacent fat stranding is much less pronounced with ischaemia vs. inflammation and may help differentiate the two in some cases.[14,21] Colonoscopy has been described as a diagnostic examination in acute colonic pseudo-obstruction in experienced hands [22] and has the added advantage of potential therapy (see below).

Key Point

- Assessment should always include a contrast study of the colon; CT is now the most commonly employed imaging method.

MANAGEMENT

Historically, acute colonic pseudo-obstruction was considered a surgical condition in which supportive therapy was, and remains a priority but in which surgery was frequently undertaken resulting in variable but usually unfavorable outcomes. Several recent advances in pharmacology and minimally invasive interventions have changed the management of this condition significantly. An algorithm, illustrating the steps and therapeutic options currently available is shown in Figure 8.2, with others published previously.[11,14,23]

Supportive Measures

Despite advances in intervention, supportive therapy is paramount in all patients even if an invasive approach is immediately necessary. Such

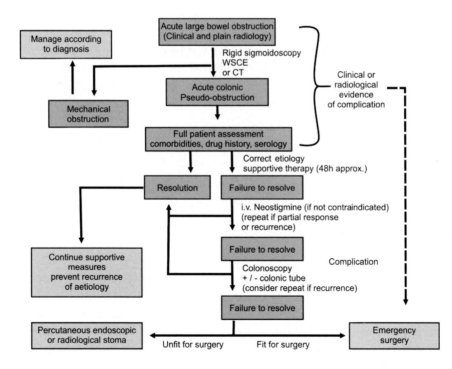

Fig. 8.2: Algorithm illustrating sequential diagnostic and treatment options for patients with acute colonic pseudo-obstruction. WSCE = water soluble contrast enema, CT = computerized tomography. Numbers = approximate percentages of patients at each stage of management.

measures should always include bowel rest, judicious intravenous fluid replacement and correction of electrolyte imbalances, especially hypokalemia and hypomagnesemia. The insertion of a rectal tube does little in reality to resolve acute colonic pseudo-obstruction but may still be effective as a supportive measure if intermittent diarrhea is problematic in a bed-bound patient. New intrarectal devices can ease nursing management in this respect and prevent pressure sores. All drugs delaying gut motility, for example opiates, anticholinergics and calcium-channel blockers, should also be avoided. Laxatives, particularly some osmotic compounds, such as lactulose are contraindicated because they may promote colonic bacterial fermentation, with the potential to increase gas production and thus luminal diameter.

If the clinical situation is not resolved after 72 hours and especially with the development of symptoms, signs and radiological features of cecal compromise, the outcome will be poor[9,11,12] unless further steps are taken. If the features of impending or actual colonic perforation have occurred then of course emergency laparotomy and colectomy are indicated. The combination of clinical findings, results of serology and sequential plain abdominal radiographs will indicate clinical course and any necessary changes in clinical direction akin to those measures employed in cases of fulminant colitis. There should be no rules concerning maximum tolerable cecal diameter viewed in isolation, but historically diameter greater than 12 cm has been considered 'at risk'.[16,17]

Success rates of conservative measures range up to 96%[24] although others report lower rates.[25] In those with failing conservative therapy but without complications, the first approach relies on pharmacological or colonoscopic decompression.

Key Point

- Patients with clinical, serological and/or radiological evidence of impending or realized cecal perforation should undergo emergency surgery.

Pharmacological Therapy

Based on the concept of parasympathetic dysfunction, intravenous neostigmine has been the only drug tested in controlled trials and remains the mainstay of drug treatment (Table 8.2).[26] Neostigmine is a reversible acetylcholinesterase inhibitor, which increases the activation of muscarinic receptors by prevention of acetylcholine breakdown, thus promoting colonic motor activity and intestinal transit. Oral administration of neostigmine is not recommended in acute colonic pseudo-obstruction because of its erratic absorption from the gastrointestinal tract.[26] Three double-blinded, randomized placebo-controlled trials have documented

TABLE 8.2

Studies using neostigmine in the treatment of acute colonic pseudo-obstruction (adapted from Knowles and de Giorgio, 2009)[14]

Study	Year	Design	N	Dose / infusion rate	Success on first dose (%)	Recurrence rate	Success on second dose (%)	Overall response (%)
Hutchinson and Griffiths	1992	P	11	2 mg, 1 min*	73	–	–	–
Stephenson et al.	1995	P	12	2·5 mg, 1–3 min	93	17	100	100
Ture´ gano-Fuentes et al.	1997	P	16	2·5 mg, 60 min	75	–	–	81
Ponec et al. [27]	1999	P RCT	11	2 mg, 3–5 min	91	27	–	64
Amaro and Rogers[28]	2000	P RCT	20	2 mg, 3–5 min	94 (17 of 18)	27	–	89 (16 of 18)
Paran et al	2000	P	11	2·5 mg, 1 h	64	22	100	82
Trevisani et al	2000	R	28	2·5 mg, 3 min	93	8	100	93
Van der Spoel et al[29]	2001	P RCT	13	0·4–0·8 mg 24 h h	85	0	–	85
Abeyta et al	2001	R	10	2-mg bolus	60	0	75	90
Loftus et al[25]	2002	R	18	2 mg, 3–5 min	89	31	–	31
Mehta et al[19]	2006	P	19	2 mg, 15 min	84	38	83	79
Sgouros et al[33]	2006	P	25	2 mg, 3–5 min	88	23	40	88

KEY: P = prospective, R = retrospective, RCT = placebo-controlled randomized controlled trial. *After guanethidine (20 mg in 100 ml saline solution) had been infused intravenously over 40 min.

the effectiveness of neostigmine.[27-29] The seminal study of Ponec et al.[27] treated 21 patients (2 mg intravenously), with the result that 10/11 (91%) under active treatment showed marked clinical and radiological improvement, whereas 10 patients in the placebo group had no response. Open-label neostigmine administration to placebo-treated patients resulted in effective decompression in seven cases. Overall, a positive response was achieved in about 94% of patients, including three patients who failed to respond to the first administration of neostigmine and eight patients in the placebo group.[27] Comparable results were obtained in two further similarly sized randomized controlled trials.[28,29] Most non-randomized studies show success rates of around 80% (Table 8.2). Other studies[19,25] have identified potential predictive factors of response to neostigmine to be female gender, advanced age and absence of anti-motility drug use.

Although neostigmine can be regarded as an effective and inexpensive tool to induce colonic decompression in acute colonic pseudo-obstruction, the use of this compound does have some significant untoward effects and contraindications. Serious side effects include bronchospasm, bradycardia and hypotension potentially leading to syncope. Therefore, during infusion, the patient's vital signs and electrocardiogram should be monitored with appropriately trained medical or paramedical support immediately on hand. Atropine should be readily available and must be promptly administered in severe cases of bradycardia. This risk can be reduced by using intravenous infusion rather than bolus or starting with a dose of 1 mg instead of 2 mg.[30] Knowledge of the spectrum of common adverse effects also predicts contraindications; caution should be exercised in patients with a history of myocardial infarction, active bronchospasm, renal failure or in those receiving treatment with β-blockers.[14,26,30] All patients should be warned that significant abdominal cramping pain frequently occurs after administration and that incontinence of flatus and liquid stool is almost inevitable.

Other potential therapies for acute colonic pseudo-obstruction have not met with equal success. Cisapride had been successfully used in some cases[31] but has now been withdrawn due to rare occurrence of severe cardiac adverse reactions. Successful outcomes with macrolide antibiotics, for example erythromycin have only been described in case reports.[32] Newer promotility agents, such as 5-HT_4 receptor agonists, for example tegaserod and prucalopride and novel peripherally acting μ-opioid receptor antagonists have yet to be tested in patients with acute colonic pseudo-obstruction.[14,26]

The role of laxatives is contentious. However, administration of polyethylene glycol (PEG) has been evaluated after initial resolution of colonic dilatation using pharmacological (neostigmine) or endoscopic decompression in a randomized placebo-controlled trial of 30 patients. Therapy with PEG resulted in a significant reduction in recurrence of cecal dilatation (33% in placebo vs. none in the PEG group), increase in bowel movements (i.e. stool and flatus evacuations), decrease in cecal, colonic diameter and reduction in abdominal circumference.[33]

> **Key Point**
>
> • In the absence of cecal compromise or medical contraindications, intravenous neostigmine is now the preferred first line therapy for acute colonic pseudo-obstruction.

ENDOSCOPIC DECOMPRESSION

Case series of colonoscopic decompression have reported success in approximately 80% of patients with acute colonic pseudo-obstruction,[34-36] although up to 20% of them may require further colonoscopy due to recurrence.[35,36] This procedure is both laborious and potentially hazardous since it is carried out on unprepared bowel. It should thus only be performed by experienced endoscopists with adequate equipment, such as colonoscopes with large diameter accessory channels for optimal suction and potential guidewire insertion. It is mandatory to deliver as little air insufflation as possible to avoid further dilatation and copious washout and suction are usually required with attendant instrument blockages and 'soiling' of the endoscopist performing the procedure. Noting the risk of perforation (approximately 2%),[36] the patient's general condition and degree of colonic dilatation should be evaluated before starting. A major benefit of colonoscopy is the ability to inspect the condition of the mucosa. When ischemia is evident, surgery will probably be required and decompression should be discontinued. On this basis, colonoscopy can also be carried out in the operating theater for patients in whom clinical features suggest that immediate surgery may be required.[17] Whether suspected ischemia is an absolute contraindication to proceed with decompression remains undecided according to an international working group.[23] Although described,[36,37] the necessity to place a colonic tube at endoscopy is debatable, given the high success rates of colonoscopy alone. Nevertheless, tube placement, usually in the right colon using guidewire and fluoroscopy is popular in the US[37] and is supported by some evidence. Two non-randomized studies showed significantly reduced rates of recurrence compared with endoscopy alone with 0/11 vs. 4/11 recurrences in one series [38] and 1/15 vs 6/14 in another.[39] Another study however suggests no difference in recurrence with or without tube placement.[40]

Percutaneous endoscopic colostomy is a minimally invasive procedure, which consists of endoscopically guided insertion of a plastic tube into the cecum or left colon, allowing decompression and irrigation. Only three studies have used this technique in pseudo-obstruction[41-43] with two

111

employing cecostomy[41,42] and one left-sided colostomy.[43] In the larger of the cecostomy series of six patients,[42] one significant complication occurred (peritonitis) but all others were successful with three remaining in place at the time of reporting. The left-sided colostomy series reported five patients with one death from peritonitis, but three successes with one remaining *in situ*. Overall success rates in the whole series of 31 with mixed indications were however tempered by a high frequency of complications.[43]

> ## Key Point
>
> - In the majority of patients unresponsive to or unsuitable for neostigmine, careful colonoscopy may effect decompression. Colonic tube placement or endoscopic colostomy should be considered if pseudo-obstruction recurs following endoscopic decompression.

Radiological Treatment

CT-guided transperitoneal percutaneous cecostomy has been reported using similar methods to those employed for other indications, for example fecal incontinence. The procedure has most commonly been applied to those patients who are unresponsive to maximal pharmacological and endoscopic therapy and also considered unfit for surgery. Except for case reports only two series of 2[44] and 5 patients[45] report data with these indicating few complications and complete resolution of colonic dilatation in all patients.[44] Larger studies will be required to fully demonstrate the efficacy and safety of this procedure and make comparisons with other interventions, including surgical decompression.

Surgery

A cautious approach should be adopted when considering surgical intervention for acute colonic pseudo-obstruction.[17] Surgery is only indicated in those with realized or imminent perforation or patients with disabling chronicity following maximum non-surgical (supportive, pharmacological and endoscopic) measures. The question of whether to proceed with surgery rather than interventional endoscopic or radiological procedures in the latter situation cannot be answered on the basis of current available data. Surgery is burdened with high morbidity and mortality rates of 30 to 60%[9,11,12] due both to the selection of complicated cases and severity of patients' medical comorbidities. If the colon is viable without perforation, the favored surgical option is some form of venting stoma with either a cecostomy or appropriate colostomy, although on table colonic tube placement has also been previously described.[11] This procedure has been performed laparoscopically in one case report.[46] Such stomas have relatively low immediate morbidity[17] but may be associated, despite claims to the contrary,[11] with both recurrence of the condition,[17] and longer term morbidity incurred by having a flush proximal, stoma that may be impossible to reverse subsequently. There are no comparable data to firmly recommend one type of stoma over another or stoma vs. resection. In the presence of complications, segmental or subtotal resection is indicated, with exteriorization[17] or extremely rarely (or perhaps never in the authors' opinion) anastomosis (ileocolic or ileorectal).

Key Point

- Surgery should be avoided if possible due to high morbidity and mortality rates. When required, stoma is almost inevitable with or without resection depending on bowel viability.

CONCLUSIONS

Acute colonic pseudo-obstruction is a life-threatening condition in which prompt diagnosis and appropriate management can limit the occurrence of complications, for example ischemia or perforation and related morbidity and mortality. Advances, particularly in pharmacological therapy, as well as those in minimally invasive endoscopic, radiological and surgical technology will no doubt improve future management and outcome.

REFERENCES

1. Bodian M, Stephens D, Ward B. Hirschsprung's disease and idiopathic megacolon. Lancet 1948;1:6.
2. Dudley HAF, Sinclair ISR, McLaren IF, et al. Intestinal pseudo-obstruction. J R Coll Surg Edin 1958;3:206-17.
3. Ogilvie WH. Large-intestine colic due to sympathetic deprivation. Br Med J 1948;2:671-3.
4. Nanni G, Garbini A, Luchetti P, et al. Ogilvie's syndrome (acute colonic pseudo-obstruction): review of the literature (October 1948 to March 1980) and report of four additional cases. Dis Colon Rectum 1982;25:157-66.
5. Stewart J, Finan PJ, Courtney DF, et al. Does a water soluble contrast enema assist in the management of acute large bowel obstruction: a prospective study of 117 cases. Br J Surg 1984;71:799-801.
6. Koruth NM, Koruth A, Matheson NA. The place of contrast enema in the management of large bowel obstruction. J R Coll Surg Edinb 1985;30:258-60.
7. Norwood MG, Lykostratis H, Garcea G, et al. Acute colonic pseudo-obstruction following major orthopaedic surgery. Colorectal Dis 2005;7:496-9.
8. Kadesky K, Purdue GF, Hunt JL. Acute pseudo-obstruction in critically ill patients with burns. Burn Care Rehabil 1995;16:132-5.
9. Vanek VW, Al-Salti M. Acute pseudo-obstruction of the colon (Ogilvie's syndrome). An analyses of 400 cases. Dis Colon Rectum 1986;29:203-10.
10. Batke M, Cappell MS. Adynamic ileus and acute colonic pseudo-obstruction. Med Clin North Am 2008;92:649-70.

11. Geelhoed GW. Colonic pseudo-obstruction in surgical patients. Am J Surg 1985;149:258-65.
12. Wegener M, Börsch G. Acute colonic pseudo-obstruction (Ogilvie's syndrome). Presentation of 14 of our own cases and analysis of 1027 cases reported in the literature. Surg Endosc 1987;1:169-74.
13. Mourelle M, Casellas F, Guarner F, et al. Induction of oxide nitric synthase in colonic smooth muscle from patients with toxic megacolon. Gastroenterology 1995;109:1497-1502.
14. Knowles CH, De Giorgio R. Acute colonic pseudo-obstruction. Br J Surg 2009; 96:229-39.
15. Sheikh RA, Yasmeen S, Pauly MP, et al. Pseudomembranous colitis without diarrhea presenting clinically as acute intestinal pseudo-obstruction. J Gastroenterol 2001;36:629-32.
16. Johnson CD, Rice RP, Kelvin FM, et al. The radiologic evaluation of gross cecal distension: emphasis on cecal ileus. Am J Roentgenol 1985;145:1211-7.
17. Williams NS. Large Bowel Obstruction. In Keighley MRB, Williams NS (Eds). Surgery of the Anus, Rectum and Colon. 1st Edition. WB Saunders: London, UK, 1997, pp 1823-66.
18. Chapman AH, McNamara M, Porter G. The acute contrast enema in suspected large bowel obstruction: value and technique. Clin Radiol 1992;46: 273-8.
19. Mehta R, John A, Nair P, et al. Factors predicting successful outcome following neostigmine therapy in acute colonic pseudo-obstruction: a prospective study. J Gastroenterol Hepatol 2006;21:459-61.
20. Beattie GC, Peters RT, Guy S, Mendelson RM. Computed tomography in the assessment of suspected large bowel obstruction. ANZ J Surg 2007;77:160-5.
21. Choi JS, Lim JS, Kim H, Choi JY, Kim MJ, Kim NK, et al. Colonic pseudoobstruction: CT findings. AJR Am J Roentgenol 2008;190:1521-6.
22. Munro A, Youngson GG. Colonoscopy in the diagnosis and treatment of colonic pseudo-obstruction. J R Coll Surg Edinb 1983;28:391-3.
23. Eisen GM, Baron TH, Dominitz JA, et al. Acute colonic pseudo-obstruction. Gastrointest Endosc 2002;56:789-92.
24. Sloyer AF, Panella VS, Demas BE, et al. Ogilvie's syndrome. Successful management without colonoscopy. Dig Dis Sci 1988;33:1391-6.
25. Loftus CG, Harewood GC, Baron TH. Assessment of predictors of response to neostigmine for acute colonic pseudo-obstruction. Am J Gastroenterol 2002;97:3118-22.
26. De Giorgio R, Barbara G, Stanghellini V, et al. Review article: The pharmacological treatment of acute colonic pseudo-obstruction. Aliment Pharmacol Ther 2001;15:1717-27.
27. Ponec RJ, Saunders MD, Kimmey MB. Neostigmine for the treatment of the acute colonic pseudo-obstruction. N Engl J Med 1999;341:137-41.
28. Amaro R, Rogers AI. Neostigmine infusion: new standard of care for acute colonic pseudo-obstruction? Am J Gastroenterol 2000;95:304-5.
29. van der Spoel JI, Oudemans-van Straaten HM, Stoutenbeek CP, et al. Neostigmine resolves critical illness-related colonic ileus in intensive care

patients with multiple organ failure: a prospective, double-blind, placebo-controlled trial. Intensive Care Med 2001;27:822-7.

30. Delgado-Aros S, Camilleri M. Pseudo-obstruction in the critically ill. Best Pract Res Clin Gastroenterol 2003;17:427-44.

31. Mac Coll C, Mac Cannell KL, Baylis B, et al. Treatment of acute colonic pseudo-obstruction(Ogilvie's syndrome) with cisapride. Gastroenterology 1990;98:773-6.

32. Armstrong DN, Ballantyne GH, Modlin IM. Erythromycin for reflex ileus in Ogilvie's syndrome. Lancet 1991;337:378.

33. Sgouros SN, Vlachogiannakos J, Vassiliadis K, et al. Effect of polyethylene glycol electrolyte balanced solution on patients with acute colonic pseudo-obstructionafter resolution of colonic dilatation: a prospective, randomized, placebo controlled trial. Gut 2006;55:638-42.

34. Kukora JS, Dent TL. Colonoscopic decompression of massive nonobstructive cecal dilation. Arch Surg 1977;112:512-7.

35. Strodel WE, Nostrant TT, Eckhauser FE, et al. Therapeutic and diagnostic colonoscopy in nonobstructive colonic dilatation. Ann Surg 1983;197:416-21.

36. Geller A, Petersen BT, Gostout CJ. Endoscopic decompression for acute colonic pseudo-obstruction. Gastrointest Endosc 1996;44:144-50.

37. Rex DK. Colonoscopy and acute colonic pseudo-obstruction. Gastrointest Endosc Clin North Am 1997;7:499-508.

38. Harig JM, Fumo DE, Loo FD, Parker HJ, Soergel KH, Helm JF, et al. Treatment of acute nontoxic megacolon during colonoscopy: tube placement versus simple decompression. Gastrointest Endosc 1988;34:23-7.

39. Lavignolle A, Jutel P, Bonhomme J, et al. Ogilvie's syndrome: results of endoscopic exsufflation in a series of 29 cases. Gastroenterol Clin Biol 1986;10:147-51.

40. Nano D, Prindiville T, Pauly M, Chow H, Ross K, Trudeau W. Colonoscopic therapy of acute pseudoobstruction of the colon. Am J Gastroenterol 1987;82:145-8.

41. Ramage JI Jr, Baron TH. Percutaneous endoscopic cecostomy: a case series. Gastrointest Endosc 2003;57:752-5.

42. Lynch CR, Jones RG, Hilden K, Wills JC, Fang JC. Percutaneous endoscopic cecostomy in adults: a case series. Gastrointest Endosc 2006;64:279-82.

43. Cowlam S, Watson C, Elltringham M, et al. Percutaneous endoscopic colostomy of the left side of the colon. Gastrointest Endosc 2007;65:1007-14.

44. Salm R, Rückauer K, Waldmann D, et al. Endoscopic percutaneous cecostomy (EPC). Surg Endosc 1988;2:92-5.

45. vanSonnenberg E, Varney RR, Casola G, et al. Percutaneous cecostomy for Ogilvie syndrome: laboratory observations and clinical experience. Radiology 1990;175:679-82.

46. Duh QY, Way LW. Diagnostic laparoscopy and laparoscopic cecostomy for colonic pseudo-obstruction. Dis Colon Rectum 1993;36:65-70.

CHAPTER NINE

Recent Advances in Surgery of Pelvic Floor Disorders

Sophie A Pilkington, Karen P Nugent

INTRODUCTION

Pelvic floor disorders are a complex group of common conditions. One in nine women will undergo surgery for pelvic floor disorders during their lifetime.[1] Of those who do undergo surgery, 30% will have additional surgery for the same condition. Unlike other branches of colorectal surgery, such as colorectal cancer and inflammatory bowel disease, there is no histological gold standard for diagnosis. Research into the underlying etiology of pelvic floor disorders has focused on collagen abnormalities,[2] but there is no unifying tissue diagnosis. Patients present with symptoms of anal incontinence, defecatory disorders, prolapse (mucosa, hemorrhoids, internal and external rectum, posterior vaginal wall (rectocele) and pelvic organ prolapse), pelvic pain and general dissatisfaction with their bowels (symptoms, such as bleeding, itching, urge fecal incontinence, passive fecal incontinence, post-defecatory leak and constipation). In the diagnosis of pelvic floor disorders it is important to exclude colorectal cancer.

The importance of a multidisciplinary team (MDT) approach to pelvic floor disorders is increasingly being recognized for both optimizing treatment[3] and for medicolegal protection.[4]

Evaluating symptoms and their impact on quality of life are key factors in managing pelvic floor patients. Investigations, including barium or MR proctography are useful to establish underlying anatomical abnormalities that may be responsible for the symptoms. Complete pelvic floor ultrasound is a new technique for evaluating patients with pelvic floor disorders.[5]

Many patients are treated conservatively with dietary modification, manipulation of stool consistency, biofeedback (BFB) and rectal irrigation. It is extremely rare for pelvic floor disorders to become life-threatening. Patients are selected for pelvic floor surgery when they have significant symptoms and when anatomical correction can be expected to relieve symptoms. An increasing number of surgical procedures have been described and these continue to be developed for treating patients with pelvic floor disorders, including sacral nerve stimulation, stapled trans anal rectal resection (STARR), laparoscopic ventral rectopexy and pelvic floor reconstruction.

PELVIC FLOOR MULTIDISCIPLINARY TEAM

The benefit of an MDT approach is well established in cancer care[6] and has recently been introduced into the management of non-malignant disorders, such as inflammatory bowel disease (IBD).[7] It has been included as one of the key standards for ensuring that IBD national health services (NHS) across the UK are able to deliver a high quality of clinical care.[8] A comprehensive pelvic floor service must also incorporate similar standards and the MDT approach.[3]

Patients with pelvic floor disorders do not have a definitive histological diagnosis and often present with a complex constellation of symptoms for which a single cause may prove elusive. Traditionally, specialists in colorectal surgery, gynecology, urology or gastroenterology have managed these patients. This organ-focused approach fails to recognize what is often a more global problem of pelvic floor dysfunction and may result in partial treatment. The impact on quality of life is easily underestimated and treatment algorithms are not as clearly established as in cancer pathways. The MDT meeting provides a forum for discussion of all these factors so that a consensus opinion can be formulated with input from all facets of the team. This is important for creating an appropriate patient-centered management plan, which has the approval of a specialist group and is aimed at improving quality of life.

Core members of the pelvic floor MDT should include:
- Colorectal surgeon with a special interest in pelvic floor disorders.
- Urogynecologist.
- Gastroenterologist with a special interest in functional bowel disorders.
- Pelvic floor practitioner and/or clinical nurse specialist and/or physiotherapist with an identified role and competency in pelvic floor disorders.
- Radiologist with a special interest in pelvic floor disorders.
- Administrative support, including database maintenance and audit.

With access to:
- Clinical psychologist
- Pain specialist

Key Point
- Pelvic floor MDT discussion of complex patients enables the establishment of a definitive management plan and is an integral component of a comprehensive pelvic floor service.

SYMPTOMS AND QUALITY OF LIFE

Patients with pelvic floor disorders present with a complex constellation of symptoms, which overlap. These include anal incontinence, defecatory disorders, pelvic pain, urinary incontinence, sexual problems and symptoms of prolapse (mucosa, hemorrhoids, internal/external rectum, posterior vaginal wall (rectocele) and pelvic organ prolapse). A detailed history and careful examination are crucial in assessing these patients. Patients are often embarrassed about their symptoms and find it difficult to explain what they are experiencing. Validated questionnaires can be used to quantify and define symptoms and assess the impact on quality of life. Two main types of questionnaire are useful for reviewing individual patient progress, auditing treatment outcomes and for research: symptom severity measures and quality of life questionnaires.

SYMPTOM SEVERITY MEASURES

Global Impression

An informal global impression of improvement is probably the most widely used measure of symptom improvement, however this is subjective. Formalizing this into a single item question (for example how does urinary incontinence after treatment compare with before treatment?) and giving the patient a choice of seven responses has been successfully validated.[9]

Patient Diaries

Two-week patient diaries to record stool frequency, incontinence episodes and straining are extremely useful at initial assessment and to monitor treatment response. Before proceeding with permanent sacral nerve stimulation (SNS), patients are asked to record their bowel habit for two weeks before and after temporary SNS wire placement. If the patient reports an improvement in symptom control and this is supported by the diaries, a permanent SNS is offered.

Symptom Severity Questionnaires

The Cleveland clinic continence score[10] is widely used but has not been rigorously validated. It is a type by frequency matrix. The maximum score is 20 and this equates to daily episodes of solid, liquid and gas anal incontinence with a daily requirement for pad usage and daily impact on lifestyle. This system is practical, simple to use and easy to interpret (Table 9.1).

The fecal incontinence severity index (FISI)[11] was described by Rockwood. It is another example of a type by frequency matrix but

TABLE 9.1

Cleveland Clinic Score for Incontinence

	Never	Rarely less than once a month	Sometimes less than once a week	Usually less than once a day	Always everyday
Solid stool leakage	0	1	2	3	4
Liquid stool leakage	0	1	2	3	4
Gas leakage	0	1	2	3	4
Pad use	0	1	2	3	4
Lifestyle restriction	0	1	2	3	4

TABLE 9.2

Rockwood's Fecal Incontinence Severity Index

	2 or more times a day	Once a day	2 or more times a week	Once a week	1 to 3 times a month	Never
a. Gas	☐	☐	☐	☐	☐	☐
b. Mucus	☐	☐	☐	☐	☐	☐
c. Liquid stool	☐	☐	☐	☐	☐	☐
d. Solid stool	☐	☐	☐	☐	☐	☐

includes patient and surgeon severity ratings depending on who is completing the questionnaire. Although well validated, this system is more complicated to use in routine practice (Table 9.2).

The patient assessment of constipation - symptom questionnaire (PAC-SYM)[12] contains 12 items and three subscales (stool, rectal and abdominal symptoms). It is a robust and reliable questionnaire.

The Bristol stool chart[13-15] uses words and pictures to describe seven stool forms (Fig. 9.1). It is valid and reproducible.

QUALITY OF LIFE QUESTIONNAIRES

Generic Questionnaires

The SF-36 questionnaire has 36 items in eight domains (physical activities, role limitations due to physical health, emotional state, bodily pain, perception of general health state, vitality, social activity and mental health).[16] It is widely used as a general measure of quality of life, although

Bristol stool chart

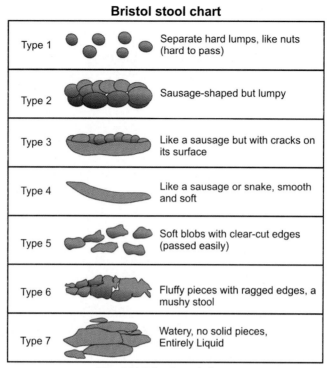

Type 1		Separate hard lumps, like nuts (hard to pass)
Type 2		Sausage-shaped but lumpy
Type 3		Like a sausage but with cracks on its surface
Type 4		Like a sausage or snake, smooth and soft
Type 5		Soft blobs with clear-cut edges (passed easily)
Type 6		Fluffy pieces with ragged edges, a mushy stool
Type 7		Watery, no solid pieces, Entirely Liquid

Fig. 9.1: Bristol stool chart.

it is less sensitive to change in pelvic floor disorders than condition specific questionnaires.[17]

Condition-Specific Questionnaires

The fecal incontinence quality of life questionnaire (FIQL) has been adopted by the American Society of Colorectal Surgeons for standard use. It contains 29 items specifically related to fecal incontinence. There are four subscales: lifestyle, coping/behavior, depression/self perception and embarrassment. It has been validated in men and women and is widely used.

The patient assessment of constipation – quality of life questionnaire (PAC-QOL)[18] contains 28 items with three subscales (worries and concerns, physical discomfort, psychosocial discomfort and satisfaction). Multinational studies have demonstrated internal consistency, reproducibility, validity and responsiveness to changes over time.

Powerful research tools are needed to define optimal treatment in pelvic floor disorders and then the same tools must be used to audit whether research results are reproducible in real life and to tailor individual treatment. Routine use of validated and reliable questionnaires is important for patients with pelvic floor disorders.

Key point

- Symptom severity and quality of life questionnaires are a useful supplement to a thorough history for the assessment of patients with pelvic floor disorders.

INVESTIGATIONS

Selection of patients for pelvic floor surgery is difficult. In general, patients are selected when surgical correction of an underlying anatomical abnormality can be expected to relieve symptoms. To evaluate the functional and anatomical abnormalities present in pelvic floor patients a wide variety of imaging modalities is available, including barium and magnetic resonance (MR) proctography and ultrasound (Figs 9.2 to 9.4).

Barium proctography is the gold standard. More recently, dynamic magnetic resonance imaging during defecation has been used. Although this avoids pelvic radiation, patients are imaged in the supine position, which is not physiological for defecation and may underestimate abnormalities. Proctography is useful for identifying patients with rectal intussusception and the degree of prolapse is described by the Oxford Grading System (Table 9.3).[19]

Endoanal 2-dimensional ultrasound is used to assess the anal sphincter for defects. Over the last decade, three-dimensional ultrasound has gained importance.[20] A technique of complete pelvic floor ultrasound has been developed using endoanal, endovaginal and transperineal probes, which allows the colorectal surgeon to assess the structure and function of the

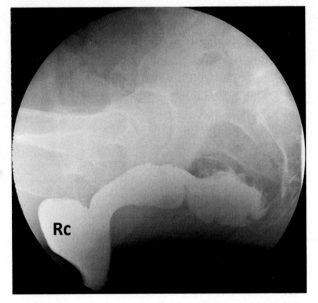

Fig. 9.2: Barium proctogram showing a rectocele (Rc).

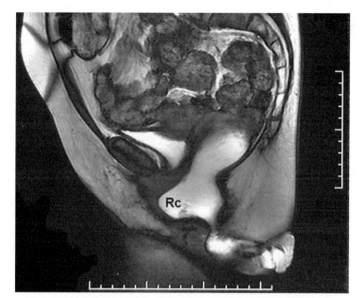

Fig. 9.3: MR proctogram showing a rectocele (Rc).

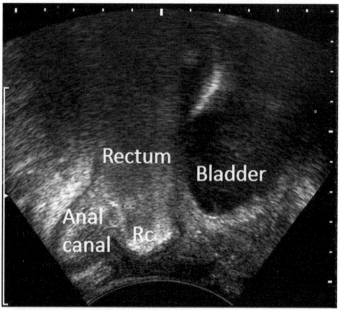

Fig. 9.4: Transperineal ultrasound showing a rectocele (Rc).

female pelvis.[5] The patient is examined in the lithotomy position and dynamic and 3-dimensional datasets are acquired. Anorectal physiology is useful in both clinical practice and research to investigate underlying causes of pelvic floor dysfunction and inform management. It is rarely used for follow-up or monitoring outcome.

TABLE 9.3

Oxford radiological grading of rectal intussusception

Grade of intussusception	Radiological characteristics of intussusceptum
I (high rectal)	Descends no lower than proximal limit of the rectocele
II (low rectal)	Descends into the level of the rectocele, but not onto sphincter/anal canal
III (high anal)	Descends onto sphincter/anal canal
IV (low anal)	Descends into sphincter/anal canal
V (overt rectal prolapse)	Protrudes from anus

Key point

- Complete pelvic floor ultrasound is a valuable addition to the physical examination in patients with pelvic floor disorders and includes three dimensional and dynamic ultrasound.

TREATMENT OPTIONS

Conservative

Dietary change and pharmacological manipulation of stool consistency may result in symptom control in patients with fecal incontinence and/or rectal evacuatory disorders.[21] Constipating agents are useful in fecal incontinence and improvements in fecal incontinence scores have been demonstrated. The Bristol Stool Chart reliably documents stool consistency and is a useful measure for monitoring patient progress and symptom control.[13-15] Rectal irrigation can be used in patients who have difficulty emptying the rectum.[22] BFB has been shown to be beneficial in the treatment of fecal incontinence with reported success rates of between 50% and 92%.[23-25] However, there are few long-term follow-up studies and a wide variety of different methods, equipment and training programs are in use. Despite the lack of high quality randomized trials,[26] BFB programs have emerged as a popular and successful treatment for fecal incontinence and a clinical improvement lasting at least two years. The method is safe, painless, well tolerated and does not preclude further treatment if it is unsuccessful.

BFB originated from psychological learning theories, such as "operant conditioning" or "task reinforcement" in the 1950s and 60s. Initially this behavioral approach was applied to all areas of medicine but cardio-vascular medicine and subsequently gastroenterology received most attention. Despite research efforts, no evidence was found to substantiate this approach in most aspects of medicine. However, over the last 30 years, a behavioral approach has been found to be useful in disorders of defecation.[27]

BFB refers to the process of amplifying a bodily function so that the individual is more aware and consequently may be able to improve function with training. In the treatment of fecal incontinence, manometric recording from the anal canal is used to provide a visual display of anal sphincter muscle activity. Most BFB programs include a series of exercises similar to pelvic floor exercises to improve muscle strength and coordination.[28] In addition to the specific techniques taught in the BFB sessions, the nurse-patient relationship is also thought to be beneficial. Fecal incontinence is an embarrassing condition, which is often difficult to verbalize (if you don't ask, they won't tell).[29] Providing the patient with a forum for discussing this problem may be therapeutic in itself and the importance of such "non-specific factors" in psychotherapy treatments is well recognized.[30] A recent study by Norton, attempted to evaluate the isolated roles of advice, advice and verbal instructions, hospital-based BFB and both hospital and home-based BFB.[24] Although over half the patients reported clinical improvement, there was no difference between the four groups and no benefit was seen with BFB. However, nurses who run the BFB services carried out this study. It is not possible to predict whether the same improvement could be achieved in a unit that does not provide BFB. Compliance with BFB programs is one of the main determinants of outcome and patients who are most likely to complete BFB are usually more severely affected, female and older than those who discontinue treatment.[31] Other factors indicative of likely success are a high level of motivation, intact cognition and absence of depression.

Key Point

- Conservative management with manipulation of stool consistency, BFB and/or rectal irrigation is usually the first line of treatment.

Neuromodulation

Stimulation of sacral nerves to improve continence, especially urinary continence, was first proposed by Brindley in the 1970s.[32] In patients in whom the spinal cord had been transected, Brindley stimulated the sacral nerves at high amplitudes and was able to demonstrate an improvement in bladder emptying. However, these levels of stimulation would be intolerable in patients with an intact spinal cord and it was not until 1992 that the present (now modified) system of sacral nerve stimulation was made commercially available in Europe. The initial studies were for urge urinary incontinence and a subgroup of patients in the initial multicenter study was seen to have an improvement in fecal continence as well. Further work was undertaken in the field of fecal incontinence, spearheaded by Cor Baeten's unit in Maastricht.

The National Institute for Clinical Excellence (NICE) reviewed the guidelines for sacral nerve stimulators in fecal incontinence in 2004 and suggested that SNS should be considered after sphincter repair.[33] However, they have updated advice on its usage in the guidelines for fecal incontinence.[34] NICE now recommends that a trial of temporary sacral nerve stimulator should be considered for people with fecal incontinence in whom sphincter surgery is deemed inappropriately. These may be patients with intact anal sphincters or those with sphincter disruption.

The trial period should last at least two weeks. The majority of units in the UK perform a trial with a percutaneous evaluation kit in which a coiled wire is passed through the sacrum onto S3 (or sometimes S2 or 4) and stimulated until there is perineal sensation (if performed under local anesthetic) or bellows movement and ipsilateral toe movement (if performed under general anesthetic).

Patients with at least 50% improvement are then considered for a permanent sacral nerve stimulator (between 50% and 75% of patients go on to have a permanent implant when tested for incontinence). The cost of the permanent procedure is around £15,000. In England and Wales, although the device is NICE supported, many primary care trusts (PCT) require a case by case application for funding. Each patient must show strict adherence to a patient pathway, maximizing medical and conservative treatment, before the PCT will consider paying for the permanent device.

The permanent device can be implanted under local or general anesthetic with the patient prone. The tyned lead is placed under image intensifier using nerve stimulation to ensure the best placement of the wires. In the NICE review, eight studies of 157 patients were reviewed for efficacy: 78% of patients improved and 24% did not; 6% had wound infections, which usually result in the removal of the implant, which can then be replaced at a later date; 18% had other complications.[34]

A European multicenter trial has recently looked at results of SNS in constipation. Of 62 patients who were recruited and trailed with a percutaneous nerve evaluation (PNE), 45 (73%) went on to have a permanent implant. There was improvement in the number of bowel actions, as well as a reduction in symptoms of constipation.[35]

Some units are now performing pudendal nerve stimulation using the same SNS kit – placing the wire directly through the buttock onto the pudendal nerve as it leaves Alcock's canal, with some promising results (personal communication – Prof Hetzer, St Gallen). As the presumed mechanism of injury in many of these patients is pudendal neuropathy following childbirth, this approach may improve the success rate of implants.

An interesting and more recent promising approach to neuromodulation is the relatively non-invasive and less expensive, posterior tibial transcutaneous nerve stimulation. An acupuncture needle is placed into the posterior tibial nerve just above the level of the ankle and stimulated for 30 minutes in one or two sessions a week.[36] Of 22 patients recruited, 18 continued treatment for more than six weeks. 13 patients had a decrease in incontinence episodes of > 50%. This is a relatively inexpensive treatment but requires intensive patient compliance and motivation.

Key Point

- Neuromodulation, most commonly as sacral nerve stimulation, has shown promising results in incontinence and constipation. It is expensive and is reserved for those in whom conservative approaches have failed.

SURGERY FOR OBSTRUCTIVE DEFECATION

Selected patients with symptoms of obstructive defecation and evidence of internal rectal prolapse on proctography are offered surgery to alleviate their symptoms. Posterior rectopexy is no longer recommended due to the poor functional outcome with many patients complaining of worsening constipation and fecal incontinence. This is probably due to the denervation of the rectum during the posterior dissection. The addition of sigmoid resection improves the functional outcome. However, the morbidity and mortality of the procedure is also increased by the presence of an anastomosis and this risk is difficult to justify when treating patients for benign disease.

Recent technological advances in laparoscopic surgery and endoanal stapling devices have contributed to the development of two new procedures for treating patients with symptomatic rectal intussusception, namely laparoscopic ventral rectopexy[37,38] and STARR.[39,40]

Key Point

- Selected patients with obstructive defecation symptoms and evidence of rectal intussusception are offered surgery in the form of laparoscopic ventral rectopexy or STARR.

An autonomic nerve-sparing laparoscopic technique for external rectal prolapse was first described by D'Hoore in 2004.[41] The long-term results are good with low recurrence rates and good function. This novel technique of laparoscopic ventral rectopexy has been extended to patients with rectal intussusception with similar effectiveness. Laparoscopic dissection takes place anterior to the rectum with preservation of the lateral ligaments. A polypropylene mesh is used for rectal fixation.[37]

Key Point

- Laparoscopic rectopexy is an autonomic nerve-sparing technique in which the anterior rectum is mobilized and fixed with mesh.

The STARR procedure (Figs 9.5 and 9.6) is a natural extension of the stapled hemorrhoidopexy. It was first described by Longo and his technique remains the gold standard. Patients treated with stapled hemorrhoidopexy, who also had symptoms of obstructive defecation, were noted to have an improvement in their obstructive symptoms as well. A reduction in distal rectal redundancy was thought to be responsible for this improvement. Stapled hemorrhoidopexy aims to eliminate mucosal and hemorrhoidal prolapse by excising a band of distal rectal mucosa at the level of the anorectal junction. This re-suspends the prolapsing tissue and reduces bleeding by interrupting the terminal branches of the superior rectal artery. In the treatment of obstructive defecation, a full thickness rectal resection is performed with a transanal stapling device. Two staple lines are placed in the anterior and posterior positions, meeting on the lateral walls of the rectum. The rectal intussusception and accompanying rectocele are removed. Relative contraindications to STARR include enterocele and poor sphincter function.[42] Serious complications have been

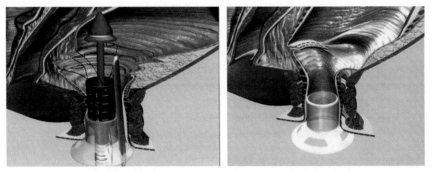

Fig. 9.5: Stapled trans anal rectal (STARR) procedure.

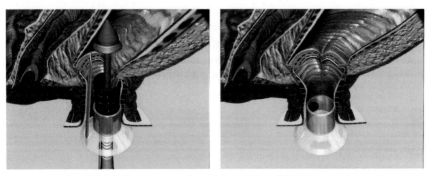

Fig. 9.6: Stapled trans anal rectal resection (STARR) procedure.

reported, including bleeding, incontinence, pain and constipation.[40] NICE issued guidelines on the use of STARR in 2006. NICE found a paucity of high quality research and concluded that the procedure should only be undertaken where there was a facility for audit and review of outcome. The UK national STARR registry was set up to meet these demands and has recently published the combined results with Germany and Italy.[39] A significant improvement in function and quality of life was demonstrated.

Key Point

- The STARR procedure involves the use of an endoanal stapling device to resect and anastomose full thickness rectum, thereby removing redundant rectum associated with rectal intussusception and rectocele.

REFERENCES

1. Kenton K, Mueller ER. The global burden of female pelvic floor disorders. BJU Int 2006;98(Suppl 1):1-5; discussion 6-7.
2. Kerkhof MH, Hendriks L, Brolmann HA. Changes in connective tissue in patients with pelvic organ prolapse—a review of the current literature. Int Urogynecol J Pelvic Floor Dysfunct 2009;20:461-74.
3. Mirnezami A, Pilkington S, Monga A, Nugent KP. Multidisciplinary team meetings for pelvic floor disorders. Colorectal Dis 2008;10:413.
4. Sidhom MA, Poulsen MG. Multidisciplinary care in oncology: medicolegal implications of group decisions. Lancet Oncol 2006;7:951-4.
5. Santoro GA, Wieczorek AP, Stankiewicz A, Wozniak MM, Bogusiewicz M, et al. High-resolution three-dimensional endovaginal ultrasonography in the assessment of pelvic floor anatomy: a preliminary study. Int Urogynecol J Pelvic Floor Dysfunct 2009;20:1213-22.
6. Ruhstaller T, Roe H, Thurlimann B, Nicoll JJ. The multidisciplinary meeting: An indispensable aid to communication between different specialities. Eur J Cancer 2006;42:2459-62.
7. Windsor A, Forbes A. Is the multidisciplinary team essential for the future management of patients with inflammatory bowel disease? Colorectal Dis 2007;9:478-9.
8. The IBD Standards Group. Quality Care: Service standards for the healthcare of people who have Inflammatory Bowel Disease (IBD): Oyster Healthcare Communications Ltd; 2009. Available from: www.ibdstandards.org.uk.
9. Yalcin I, Bump RC. Validation of two global impression questionnaires for incontinence. Am J Obstet Gynecol 2003;189:98-101.
10. Jorge JM, Wexner SD. Etiology and management of fecal incontinence. Dis Colon Rectum 1993;36:77-97.
11. Rockwood TH, Church JM, Fleshman JW, Kane RL, Mavrantonis C, et al. Patient and surgeon ranking of the severity of symptoms associated with fecal incontinence: the fecal incontinence severity index. Dis Colon Rectum 1999;42:1525-32.

12. Frank L, Kleinman L, Farup C, Taylor L, Miner P, Jr. Psychometric validation of a constipation symptom assessment questionnaire. Scand J Gastroenterol 1999;34:870-7.

13. Heaton KW, Ghosh S, Braddon FE. How bad are the symptoms and bowel dysfunction of patients with the irritable bowel syndrome? A prospective, controlled study with emphasis on stool form. Gut 1991;32:73-9.

14. Heaton KW, Radvan J, Cripps H, Mountford RA, Braddon FE, et al. Defecation frequency and timing, and stool form in the general population: a prospective study. Gut 1992;33:818-24.

15. O'Donnell LJ, Virjee J, Heaton KW. Detection of pseudodiarrhoea by simple clinical assessment of intestinal transit rate. BMJ 1990;300:439-40.

16. Ware JE, Jr., Sherbourne CD. The MOS 36-item short-form health survey (SF-36). I. Conceptual framework and item selection. Med Care 1992;30:473-83.

17. Rockwood TH, Church JM, Fleshman JW, Kane RL, Mavrantonis C, et al. Fecal Incontinence Quality of Life Scale: quality of life instrument for patients with fecal incontinence. Dis Colon Rectum 2000;43:9-16; discussion-7.

18. Marquis P, De La Loge C, Dubois D, McDermott A, Chassany O. Development and validation of the Patient Assessment of Constipation Quality of Life questionnaire. Scand J Gastroenterol 2005;40:540-51.

19. Collinson R, Cunningham C, D'Costa H, Lindsey I. Rectal intussusception and unexplained fecal incontinence: findings of a proctographic study. Colorectal Dis 2009;11:77-83.

20. Gold DM, Bartram CI, Halligan S, Humphries KN, Kamm MA, et al. Three-dimensional endoanal sonography in assessing anal canal injury. Br J Surg 1999;86:365-70.

21. Lauti M, Scott D, Thompson-Fawcett MW. Fibre supplementation in addition to loperamide for fecal incontinence in adults: a randomized trial. Colorectal Dis 2008;10:553-62.

22. Gardiner A, Marshall J, Duthie G. Rectal irrigation for relief of functional bowel disorders. Nurs Stand 2004;19:39-42.

23. Solomon MJ, Pager CK, Rex J, Roberts R, Manning J. Randomized, controlled trial of biofeedback with anal manometry, transanal ultrasound, or pelvic floor retraining with digital guidance alone in the treatment of mild to moderate fecal incontinence. Dis Colon Rectum 2003;46:703-10.

24. Norton C, Chelvanayagam S, Wilson-Barnett J, Redfern S, Kamm MA. Randomized controlled trial of biofeedback for fecal incontinence. Gastroenterology 2003;125:1320-9.

25. Norton C, Kamm MA. Outcome of biofeedback for fecal incontinence. Br J Surg 1999;86:1159-63.

26. Pares D, Norton C, Chelvanayagam S. Fecal incontinence: the quality of reported randomized, controlled trials in the last ten years. Dis Colon Rectum 2008;51:88-95.

27. Enck P, Van der Voort IR, Klosterhalfen S. Biofeedback therapy in fecal incontinence and constipation. Neurogastroenterol Motil 2009;21:1133-41.

28. Norton C, Chelvanayagam S. Methodology of biofeedback for adults with fecal incontinence: a program of care. J Wound Ostomy Continence Nurs 2001;28:156-68.

29. Whitehead WE. Diagnosing and managing fecal incontinence: if you don't ask, they won't tell. Gastroenterology 2005;129:6.

30. Chelvanayagam S, Stern J. Using therapeutic groups to support women with fecal incontinence. Br J Nurs 2007;16:214-8.

31. Byrne CM, Solomon MJ, Young JM, Rex J, Merlino CL. Biofeedback for fecal incontinence: short-term outcomes of 513 consecutive patients and predictors of successful treatment. Dis Colon Rectum 2007;50:417-27.

32. Brindley GS. Emptying the bladder by stimulating sacral ventral roots. J Physiol 1974;237:15P-6P.

33. National Institute for Health and Clinical Excellence. Sacral nerve stimulation for fecal incontinence: IPG99. London: National Institute for Health and Clinical Excellence; 2004.

34. National Institute for Health and Clinical Excellence. Fecal incontinence: the management of fecal incontinence in adults. CG49. London: National Institute for Health and Clinical Excellence; 2007.

35. Dudding T. Sacral Nerve Stimulation for Bowel Dysfunction: Improving Outcomes and expanding indications. London: University of London; 2009.

36. Govaert B, Pares D, Delgado-Aros S, La Torre F, van Gemert W, et al. A Prospective Multicenter Study to investigate Percutaneous Tibial Nerve Stimulation for the Treatment of Fecal Incontinence. Colorectal Dis 2009.

37. Slawik S, Soulsby R, Carter H, Payne H, Dixon AR. Laparoscopic ventral rectopexy, posterior colporrhaphy and vaginal sacrocolpopexy for the treatment of recto-genital prolapse and mechanical outlet obstruction. Colorectal Dis 2008;10:138-43.

38. Collinson R, Wijffels N, Cunningham C, Lindsey I. Laparoscopic ventral rectopexy for internal rectal prolapse: Short-term functional results. Colorectal Dis 2009.

39. Jayne DG, Schwandner O, Stuto A. Stapled transanal rectal resection for obstructed defecation syndrome: one-year results of the European STARR Registry. Dis Colon Rectum 2009;52:1205-12; discussion 12-4.

40. Dodi G, Pietroletti R, Milito G, Binda G, Pescatori M. Bleeding, incontinence, pain and constipation after STARR transanal double stapling rectotomy for obstructed defecation. Tech Coloproctol 2003;7:148-53.

41. D'Hoore A, Cadoni R, Penninckx F. Long-term outcome of laparoscopic ventral rectopexy for total rectal prolapse. Br J Surg 2004;91:1500-5.

42. Schwandner O, Stuto A, Jayne D, Lenisa L, Pigot F, et al. Decision-making algorithm for the STARR procedure in obstructed defecation syndrome: position statement of the group of STARR Pioneers. Surg Innov 2008;15: 105-9.

CHAPTER TEN

Laparoscopic Total Mesorectal Excision (TME) for Rectal Cancer

Anil Hemandas, Daniel O' Leary, Amjad Parvaiz

The development of laparoscopic surgery provided a major opportunity to improve the management of colorectal cancer in the last two decades. Laparoscopic surgery for the colon was first reported in 1991.[1] Today, laparoscopic surgery for colon cancer has been well proven by randomized studies to benefit patients: the procedure results in earlier recovery of bowel function, reduced blood loss, less postoperative pain and decreased hospital stay compared with conventional open colectomy.[2-5] Most of these studies have also shown adequate lymph node yields and tumor clearance in addition to the superior short-term outcomes in terms of reduced postoperative pain, shorter hospital stay, reduced ileus and comparable long-term outcomes.[6] While the minimally invasive approach for colonic resections has become well established and accepted, its role in the management of rectal cancer is still evolving.

Key Point

- Laparoscopic surgery for colon cancer has been well proven by randomized studies to benefit patients with better postoperative outcomes and comparable long-term oncologic outcomes.

RECTAL RESECTION WITH TME: DEVELOPMENT OF A GOLD STANDARD

In the early 20th century, the local recurrence rate following surgery for rectal cancer was nearly 100%. This fell to 30% after the introduction of Miles' operation - a combined radical abdominal and perineal approach to remove the rectum and the "zone of upward spread" along the superior hemorrhoidal and inferior mesenteric arteries.[7]

The concept of total mesorectal excision (TME) during rectal anterior resection was introduced by Heald in 1979.[8] The goal of TME is the excision of the rectum along with its blood vessels and surrounding lymph nodes within an intact visceral fascial envelope. Preserving the integrity of this mesorectal fascial envelope and obtaining a negative circumferential margin are the key elements in minimizing pelvic recurrence. Later refinements included preservation of the pelvic autonomic nerves and nerve plexuses. Heald reported rates of local recurrence as low as 2.7% after potentially curative resection for rectal cancer. He simultaneously showed that it was possible to perform a restorative resection in as many as 90% of rectal cancers with a permanent stoma rate of less than 10%. Nonetheless, such major pelvic dissection with low colorectal or coloanal anastomosis has been associated with considerable morbidity. Anastomotic leak rates of > 15% have been commonly reported and most TME surgeons advocate temporary defunctioning of these anastomoses in order to reduce the consequences if not the frequency of anastomotic leakage.[9]

Heald's results from Basingstoke stimulated the surgical community and led to training programs in TME within the UK and internationally. Several series have now reported successful application of TME principles with reduction in local recurrence rates to < 10%. Low anterior resection with TME has become the gold standard in the surgical management of rectal cancer.[10-11]

Key Point

- Using total mesorectal excision (TME) for rectal cancer can achieve rates of local recurrence well below 10%.

LAPAROSCOPIC TME

Laparoscopic anterior resection was first described in the early 1990s. However, even with pioneering surgeons, laparoscopic operating low in the pelvis was challenging, owing to the technical limitations of the available equipment. It would have been difficult for these initial operations to achieve oncologic equivalence with optimal conventional TME surgery. High conversion rates, postoperative morbidity and significant port site and local recurrence rates, all inhibited the wider adoption of laparoscopic resection for rectal cancer.[12]

Since then, advances in laparoscopic instrumentation and imaging technology together with improved tools for dissecting, hemostasis and anastomosis, coupled with increased surgical skill, training and experience have led to several reports of successful laparoscopic resections of rectal cancer with TME and increasing evidence that this is now appropriate management.

Potential Advantages of Laparoscopic TME

1. **More precise anatomical TME dissection:** No part of a laparoscopic TME need to be completely blind, a 30° camera allows a clear view even low in the pelvis. By contrast, conventional TME dissection, especially low posteriorly in a male pelvis is often difficult to complete

under direct vision. The laparoscopic view is also well illuminated and magnified making it easier to see and follow surgical planes.

2. **Reduced trauma to the oncologic specimen with less inadvertent compromise of specimen quality:** Laparoscopic operating tends to displace the rectum and mesorectum gently from side to side. The laparoscope can operate in a very confined space and illuminates its view. In contrast, considerable traction is required to obtain lighting and a view low in the pelvis in conventional resection. Such handling and retraction of the oncologic specimen can cause tears into the mesorectum or even into the lumen. Once a tear begins, it tends to progress because traction on the specimen is difficult to avoid during open operations. Rates of R0 resection might be higher following laparoscopic resection.

3. **Faster postoperative recovery:** Laparoscopic resection offers the potential for reduced blood transfusion requirements, reduced surgical trauma, a less marked inflammatory response, earlier return of gut function and shorter hospital stay compared with conventional operating.

Key Point

- Improvements in image quality and better instrumentation coupled with increasing experience should lead to more precise dissection and hence better short- and long-term outcomes.

Published Evidence Concerning the Oncologic Quality and Outcome of Laparoscopic Anterior Resection with TME

Many studies reporting laparoscopic TME include small numbers of patients and follow-up of less than 3 years. In addition, some studies that claim to have performed TME have not consistently provided information regarding height of tumor from the anal verge, oncological data, such as distance from distal margin, clearance of circumferential margin and selection/exclusion criteria.[13-15]

By contrast, Bretagnol et al reported a prospective series of 144 laparoscopic TMEs with low colorectal or coloanal anastomosis for mid and low rectal cancers of stage T3 N1 or less.[16] Their conversion rate was 14%. Clear distal and circumferential margins were achieved in 98% and 94% respectively. Two patients developed local recurrence and the 3-year overall and disease-free survival rates were 89 and 77% respectively.

Zhou et al reported excellent results of laparoscopic resection for rectal cancer with TME and sphincter preservation in their randomized trial.[17] Their overall morbidity rate was 6.1%, anastomotic leakage rate was 1.2%, mean operative blood loss was 20 ml and mean operating time was 120 min. However, the report provided no details on the method of randomization or definition and the rate of conversion, nor whether the analysis was performed on an intention-to-treat basis.

Lujan et al from Murcia, Spain have reported a single center randomized controlled trial (RCT) in which 204 patients with mid and low rectal cancers were randomized between open and laparoscopic resection.[18] Patients in the laparoscopic group had mean return of gut function and hospital stay of 2.8 days and 8.2 days respectively but this was not significantly different from the open group. There were fewer anastomotic leaks in the laparoscopic group, circumferential resection margin (CRM) positivity was 4%, five-year local recurrence was 4.8%, disease free survival was 84.8% and overall survival 72.1%. Overall, the results demonstrated oncological equivalence with decreased transfusion requirements following laparoscopic resection.

The conventional versus laparoscopic-assisted surgery in colorectal cancer (CLASICC) trial offers substantial evidence on laparoscopic resection for rectal cancer.[19-20] It included patients with colorectal cancers from 27 centers in the UK and provided detailed subgroup analysis of short- and long-term outcomes of patients with rectal cancer. 242 laparoscopic rectal resections were performed, in which 129 were TMEs. The benefits with laparoscopic surgery of lower intraoperative blood loss, less pain, early return of gut function and less narcotic use were confirmed. Hospital stay was 11 days and was shorter than the 13 days for open TME group. This trial has been criticized for high conversion rates of 34% and high rates of CRM positivity of 16%. A subsequent three years update of outcomes in this trial revealed equivalent oncologic and quality of life outcomes for the laparoscopic and open groups (overall survival 74.6% laparoscopic and 66.7% open, $p = 0.17$). In addition, the trend toward increased CRM positivity seen in the laparoscopic group did not result in an increased rate of local recurrence (7.8% laparoscopic and 7.0% open, $p = 0.70$) and the administration of neoadjuvant chemoradiation and adjuvant chemotherapy was equivalent in both groups.

The inclusion criteria for the CLASICC trial were for the operating surgeons to have performed > 20 laparoscopic resections before submitting patients onto the trial. It has been suggested that the learning curve may actually be bimodal, with improvement continuing to > 100 cases.[21] It is possible therefore that the outcomes could be better for surgeons with more experience with laparoscopic rectal cancer surgery.

A recent systematic review and meta-analysis comparing short- and medium-term outcomes of over 1,400 laparoscopic versus 1,755 open TMEs concluded that there were no oncological differences between laparoscopic and open resections for the treatment of primary rectal cancer.[22]

Laurent et al emphasized the importance of specialization in TME in their series of 238 laparoscopic TMEs with 5-year follow-up (median follow-up = 52 months).[23] More than 80% of their rectal resections were for mid and low tumors. All patients were treated with curative intent.

Their conversion rate was 15%. The local recurrence rate was 3.8% in laparoscopic completed and no worse (3.5%) in laparoscopic converted cases both these figures being lower than the 5.5% observed for their open TMEs. These results are in line with the observations of other groups[24-26] showing that adequately trained laparoscopic surgeons can obtain equivalent long-term oncologic results to open TME surgeons.

Additionally, a notable observation made by Laurent et al was that the overall survival at 5 years was better in the laparoscopic group than in the open group, especially in Stage III cancers. Similar observations have been reported by Morino et al and Strohlein et al for stage III rectal cancers and by Lacy et al for stage III colon cancers.[27-29] This possible advantage of laparoscopic surgery for survival requires further investigation.

These reports from surgeons and centers at the leading edge of developments in laparoscopic colorectal cancer surgery show that laparoscopic resection for rectal cancer with TME can be achieved without oncologic compromise and with potential benefits in terms of transfusion requirements, return of gut function, R0 resection rates and length of stay when compared to conventional resection (Tables 10.1 and 10.2).

Key Point

- Published evidence suggests better short-term outcomes with low local recurrence rates and comparable five-year survival between laparoscopic and open TME surgery.

Morbidity and Mortality of Laparoscopic TME Surgery

Rectal cancer resections are generally associated with substantial rates of morbidity and mortality. Several large published series of laparoscopic TME and experience in our unit show an overall mortality rate of about 1 to 2% which compares favorably with the 3 to 8% range reported in open surgery[30] and postoperative morbidity ranging between 18 and 37% (Table 10.1).

Anastomotic Leaks

Some of the large series have reported leak rates ranging from 10 to 17% after laparoscopic TME. However, with increasing experience, anastomotic leak rates appear to be declining. In a case-control study comparing laparoscopic and open TME, Breukink et al reported 9% anastomotic leakage in the laparoscopic group vs 14% in the open group.[31] Lujan et al in their recently published single center randomized trial of laparoscopic versus open TMEs for mid and low rectal cancers, reported anastomotic leak rates of 6% in the laparoscopic group as against 12% in the open TME group.[18] Similarly, Tsang et al from Hong Kong had only 1 anastomotic leak in their series of 105 laparoscopic **135**

TABLE 10.1

Studies reporting on early outcomes after laparoscopic surgery for rectal cancer

Author or trial name	n*	Median tumor height (cm)	Conversion (%)	CRM + (%)	Leak (%)	Other morbidity (%)	Mortality (%)	Median LOS (range)	Re-admission (%)	Re-operation (%)
RANDOMIZED STUDIES										
Zhou[17]	82	(1.5-8)	—	0	1.2	6	—	8 (5-11)	—	—
Guillou[3] (CLASICC)	131	—	34	16	10	59	4	11 (9-15)	—	—
NON-RANDOMIZED STUDIES										
Rezvani[56]	46	—	16	—	—	7	2	4	—	2
Strohlen[28]	114	—	22	4	10	10	0	15 (8-59)	—	—
Laurent[42]	200	2.5 (0.5-8)	15.5	11	8	25	1	9 (4-42)	—	—
Tjandra[57]	31	2.6 (1.8-3.4)	35	3.2	0	25	0	6	—	0
Lelong[55]	104	—	14.5	9	11.5	43	1	10 (4-72)	—	8
Staudacher[43]	202	6.2 (4.2-8.2)	6	2.6	17	32	0	10 (6-14)	—	6
Breukink[31]	41	10	10	7	9	37	0	11 (6-50)	—	12
Portsmouth (unpublished)	106	8 (2-10)	3.7	1.8	0.9	—	0.9	6 (2-50)	18	2

*= only TMEs are included; LOS = Length of stay

TABLE 10.2

Studies reporting on long-term outcomes after laparoscopic surgery for rectal cancer

Author or trial name	n	Median follow-up (months)	Local recurrence (%)	Overall Survival (%)	Disease-Free Survival (%)
RANDOMIZED STUDIES					
Jayne (CLASICC)[20]	131	36 (20-61.5)	9.7	74.6 (3 yr)	70.9 (3 yr)
Lujan[18]	101	34.1 (14-54)	4.8	72.1	84.8
Staudacher[43]	202	40	6.1	81	70
Lee[59]	326	29 (6-92)	9.5	—	—
NON-RANDOMIZED STUDIES					
Laurent[22]	238	52 (1-151)	3.8	83	83
Bianchi[60]	107	36	1	81.4	79.8
Braga[61]	83	54	4 (3 yr)	—	—
Morino[24]	87	45.7 (12-72)	4.2	74	63
Leroy[26]	89	36	6	65	—
Tsang[25]	105	26.9 (1.3-65.6)	8.9	76.9	64.4
Bretagnol[16]	144	18 (1-46)	1.4 (3 yr)	89 (3 yr)	77 (3 yr)
Ng[44]	151	56 (8-188)	4.6	70	—
Kim[58]	257	30 (8-68)	2.9	—	—

rectal cancer resections.[25] Results in our own unit are in agreement with these figures (unpublished data) with a leak rate of 0.9% following laparoscopic TME (n = 106) as against 3.3% (n = 60) after conventional TME.

Autonomic Nerve Damage

Laparoscopic TME has the potential to achieve better preservation of the pelvic autonomic nerves because the magnified operative view allows easier identification of pelvic nerves. Liang et al studied 98 patients with T3 mid or low rectal cancers undergoing laparoscopic TME following neo-adjuvant chemo-radiotherapy.[32] Patients underwent pre and postoperative assessment of urinary and sexual function using a standardized questionnaire. Any patients with abnormal urinary or sexual function preoperatively were excluded. They reported that it was possible for the majority of their patients to retain satisfactory genitourinary function following a laparoscopic TME with autonomic nerve preservation (ANP) technique. Similarly, Asoglu et al, in their series of 34 laparoscopic and

29 open TMEs, found that the open technique was associated with a significantly higher incidence of sexual dysfunction, but not bladder dysfunction compared with laparoscopic TME. [33]

However, Jayne et al in the only randomized trial investigating genitourinary function after laparoscopic TME, found worse overall sexual and erectile function in men undergoing laparoscopic TME than after open TME (p = 0.063 and 0.068 respectively).[34] There was no difference in urinary function between the two groups and in both sexes. These results may be due to the learning curve associated with the technique. Further randomized studies are expected to help address this matter conclusively.

Key Point

- Laparoscopic TME surgery is associated with very low mortality and low anastomotic leak rates with similar preservation of pelvic autonomic nerve function to open surgery.

IMPLEMENTATION OF A TRAINING PROGRAM IN LAPAROSCOPIC RECTAL RESECTION WITH TME

Surgeon Selection and Training

Laparoscopic rectal resection with TME requires advanced laparoscopic skills, a secure grounding in conventional TME techniques, a good understanding of surgical oncological principles as applied to rectal cancer and an appropriate preceptored training in laparoscopic TME. Technically, this is a challenging surgery. It requires intense concentration over a prolonged period, sequential operating in several surgical fields and meticulous technique to achieve a perfect TME.

Martling and Heald showed that local recurrence rates decreased by more than 50% as a result of a surgical teaching initiative for open TME in Stockholm.[35] A similar approach is likely to be required to fulfil the training needs of surgeons who have gained competency with laparoscopic colonic surgery and wish to embark upon laparoscopic TME surgery for rectal cancer. Since laparoscopic surgery allows the procedure to be monitored and recorded, it can also be used as a learning tool outside the operating theater. We strongly recommend that laparoscopic TME surgery should be performed after closely supervised training and with ongoing audit of clinical and oncologic results in a manner comparable to the open TME training project.[36]

Whereas laparoscopic resection for colon cancer may be genaralizable to a wide pool of colorectal surgeons, this is much less likely with laparoscopic resection for rectal cancer. Many colorectal surgeons can perform a satisfactory conventional TME but few will be able to carry out a laparoscopic version of the same surgery. As minimally invasive surgery takes hold it is likely that laparoscopic management of rectal cancer will be concentrated increasingly in the hands of a small number of colorectal surgeons and perhaps in a small number of specialist centers.

Laparoscopic Total Mesorectal Excision (TME) for Rectal Cancer

Key Point

- Training programs similar to those used for open TME need to be implemented for laparoscopic TME with an ongoing commitment to audit surgical and oncologic outcomes in all units undertaking this surgery.

Patient Selection

Patients with significant comorbidity, high BMI, locally advanced cancers or who have undergone preoperative long course downstaging chemo-radiotherapy all present distinct challenges with regard to rectal cancer surgery. Some surgeons believe that such patients are better managed by conventional surgery and exclude them from laparoscopic surgery.[37-38] Patients with cardio-respiratory comorbidity and high ASA grade benefit from quick rather than prolonged operations and may be adversely affected by head down tilt and pneumoperitoneum. However, such patients are also likely to benefit from the faster recovery afforded by laparoscopic resection. We have found that this group of patients benefits overall from laparoscopic rectal resection with reduced rates of complications and shorter hospital stay versus conventional resection.[39]

Obesity with high BMI, locally advanced cancers and previous long course radiotherapy all increase the difficulty in completing rectal resection with TME whether laparoscopic or conventional.[40-41] However, we have shown that these cases can be offered laparoscopic resection with similar outcomes to more traditionally favorable groups.[39]

Patients with locally advanced rectal cancers who require multivisceral resection or where the bulk of the tumor is large, may not have much to gain from a laparoscopic pelvic dissection. However, in progressive colorectal units, this will be a relatively small proportion of all rectal cancers.

Conversion to Open Surgery

Conversion rates range widely between 1.9% and 34%.[3, 24-26] The most common reasons cited for conversion include technical difficulties secondary to tumor fixity, dense adhesions or inadequate visualization due to obesity, uncertainties regarding the oncological completeness or hemorrhage. It has also been suggested by Laurent et al that male sex and stapled anastomosis are independent risk factors for conversion.[42] However, the definition of conversion in laparoscopic rectal surgery has varied between authors with some describing hybrid operations in which the rectum is mobilized by an open technique where others would consider these as conversions.[25, 43-44] We believe that the need to use an open technique to mobilize the rectum during any part of the laparoscopic TME should be regarded as a conversion.

The experience of the operating surgeon is a major determinant of the conversion rate. Conversion rates have generally decreased over recent years, attributable to a combination of improved instrumentation, imaging technology, increasing experience and perhaps better patient selection. Tsang et al had two conversions in 105 laparoscopic TMEs and Leroy et al in their series of 102 laparoscopic TMEs involving patients across all T stages reported a conversion rate of 3%.[25-26] The conversion rate in our unit for laparoscopic TME surgery is 3.7% with satisfactory oncological outcomes (unpublished data).

Conversion Should not Compromise Oncologic Outcomes

A German prospective study found an association between high conversion rates and poor oncological outcome in terms of local recurrence.[28] In their study of 389 patients, 114 laparoscopic rectal resections were attempted. There were 25 conversions (21.9%). Of the 89 laparoscopic completed resections, 47.2% were TMEs. The local recurrence rate was 16% in the converted group as against 6.9 and 9.5% in the laparoscopic completed and the open group respectively. The main reasons for conversion were tumor fixity and rectal perforation. It is interesting to note that 76% of the conversions ($n = 19$) occurred within the first half of the inclusion period between 1998 and 2001, reflecting the learning curve of the operating surgeons. The other possible explanation for this could be that these very locally advanced tumors necessitating conversions had an unfavorable outlook, which increased local recurrence rates.

It is likely that conversion will not increase local recurrence rates, provided the decision to convert is made before there is any compromise of resection planes or resection margins (as may have happened in the German study above). A misguided laparoscopic "trial dissection" that compromises an oncological resection that would have been straightforward if performed conventionally may condemn the patient to an avoidable R1 resection with local recurrence and should be avoided. It is more important to complete the operation in an oncologically sound and radical manner than to complete it laparoscopically.

> ## Key Point
> - Conversion to open surgery should not compromise either clinical or oncological outcomes provided the decision is made before any compromise of resection planes or margins.

Low Rectal Division and Anastomosis

Conventional cross-stapled anastomosis is more difficult to achieve laparoscopically than in open surgery because the available staplers for laparoscopic use are not able to flex sufficiently to allow easy placement of a staple line across the rectum at right angles. Frequently, it is necessary to use a number of firings of the stapler to transect the rectum along a more oblique line than intended.

Indeed, Leroy et al in an attempt to explain their 17% clinical leak rate, hypothesized that such a long staple line increases the risk of leakage.[26] They postulated that refinement of the staplers and the technique of stapling, in order to enable the stapling device to be applied at a right angle to the bowel, would result in a short staple line and a potential reduction in the leak rate. Brannigan et al examined the technique of laparoscopic rectal stapling following TME using a virtual model and simulation of laparoscopic stapling. They concluded that the minimal angulation of the stapler head required for successful transverse stapling of the rectum was 62 to 68°.[45]

For adequate clearance below a low rectal cancer a transverse rather than an oblique transection of the rectum is optimal. In order to compensate for the limited angulation of current laparoscopic staplers it is necessary to employ special techniques to ensure adequate clearance and safe anastomosis for very low rectal cancers. These include:
1. Perineal pressure to render the lowest part of the rectum more accessible for staple-transection.
2. Dissection into the pelvic funnel in the intersphincteric plane to allow the somewhat oblique staple line to adequately clear the low neoplasm.
3. Transanal division of the rectum and hand-sutured coloanal anastomosis.

Routine or Selective Use of Defunctioning Stomas

Distal colorectal and coloanal anastomoses are defunctioned to prevent serious morbidity and reduce the likelihood of a permanent stoma if the anastomosis leaks. It is our practice to routinely defunction following laparoscopic TME for mid to low rectal cancer (our anastomotic leak rate is 1.1%). However, defunctioning stomas cause morbidity and closure carries a significant rate of complications. If leak rates are low (e.g. < 2% versus > 15% for open surgery) a case could be made to defunction more selectively, typically for more and more distal anastomoses only.

Routine or Selective Mobilization of the Splenic Flexure

Laparoscopic mobilization of the splenic flexure adds to operative time, adds a (small) potential for splenic injury and may be unnecessary. Experience in open surgery suggests that use of the sigmoid colon for colorectal or coloanal anastomosis is safe.[46] Data from our unit suggest that following laparoscopic anterior resection for low rectal cancers, the sigmoid may be safely preserved, perfused on the marginal arcade and that by so doing a low anastomosis may be safely performed with low rates of leakage without routinely mobilizing the splenic flexure.

ROBOTIC SURGERY

The first robotic laparoscopic colectomy was reported by Weber et al in 2001.[47] Since then, a wide range of colorectal operations has been performed robotically, initially for benign diseases[48] and later for malignant disease,[49-50] with short-term and oncological outcomes comparable to laparoscopy.

Full robotic and robotic-assisted surgery overcomes the technical difficulties in complex and difficult laparoscopic surgery by providing tri-dimensional imaging and instruments with seven degrees of freedom that mimic hand movements and dexterity. It also eliminates hand tremors, which further enhances precision.[51]

A very low conversion rate for robotic colorectal operations has been reported, with total mesorectal excision in a narrow pelvis, identification of the hypogastric plexus, dissection of the inferior mesenteric vessels and mobilization of the splenic flexure.[52] However, many authors still prefer to use a hybrid technique and take advantage of the robotic precise dissection only during the total mesorectal excision. A disadvantage of robotic dissection is that multiquadrant operation for left colonic resection increases operative time as the robotic cart has to be moved twice.

Despite its potential advantages, robotic TME surgery is not established as standard practice and issues, such as hybrid operations, (laparoscopy with robotic surgery), second intervention, conversion, cost, standardization of technique and training will have to be addressed before its use can become widespread. A RCT is also required to establish the efficacy or superiority of this approach over the existing techniques prior to its wider introduction.

Key Point

- Robots provide freedom of 360° movements and three dimensional high quality images. Cost and availability may be the rate limiting steps for greater uptake of this technique.

CONCLUSION

Laparoscopic TME is a technically demanding procedure. After initial hesitation regarding oncological safety and technical feasibility, increasing experience and better instrumentation have enabled progressive uptake of this technique by experienced laparoscopic colorectal surgeons. Most of the evidence for laparoscopic TME is from prospective or retrospective case series; it weighs heavily in favor of the laparoscopic approach.

Currently, two major multicenter RCTs are being conducted in the Europe and the United States: the COLOR II trial and the ACOSOG - Z6051, respectively.[53-54] Both these trials are designed to compare laparoscopic versus open resection for curable rectal cancer and it is envisaged that their results will provide vital information regarding the practice of laparoscopic rectal cancer surgery.

Key Point

- Increasing evidence suggests that laparoscopic TME surgery is rapidly becoming the new gold standard for rectal cancer management in specialist units. Two large RCTs currently underway should provide long-term data on oncological outcomes.

REFERENCES

1. Jacobs M, Verdeja JC, Goldstein HS. Minimally invasive colon resection (laparoscopic colectomy). Surg Laparosc Endosc 1991;1:144-50.
2. Lacy AM, Garcia-Valdecasas JC, Delgado S, et al. Laparoscopy-assisted colectomy versus open colectomy for treatment of non-metastatic colon cancer: a randomised trial. Lancet 2002;359:2224-9.
3. Guillou PJ, Quirke P, Thorpe H, et al. Short-term endpoints of conventional versus laparoscopic-assisted surgery in patients with colorectal cancer (MRC CLASICC trial): multicentre randomised controlled trial. Lancet 2005;365: 1718-26.
4. Clinical Outcomes of Surgical Therapy Study Group. A comparison of laparoscopically assisted and open colectomy for colon cancer. N Engl J Med 2004;350:2050-9.
5. Veldkamp R, Kuhry E, Hop WC, et al. Laparoscopic surgery versus open surgery for colon cancer: short-term outcomes of a randomised trial. Lancet Oncol 2005;6:477-84.
6. Fleshman J, Sargent DJ, Green E, Anvari M, et al. Laparoscopic colectomy for cancer is not inferior to open surgery on 5-year data from the COST Study Group trial. Ann Surg 2007;246:655-62.
7. Miles WE. A method of performing abdomino-perineal resection for carcinoma of the rectum and of the terminal portion of the pelvic colon. Lancet 1908;2: 1812-3.
8. Heald RJ. A new approach to rectal cancer. Br J Hosp Med 1979;22:277-81.
9. Matthiessen P, Hallbook O, Rutegard J, Simert G, Sjodahl R. Defunctioning stoma reduces symptomatic anastomotic leakage after low anterior resection of the rectum for cancer: a randomized multicenter trial. Ann Surg 2007; 246:207-14.
10. MacFarlane JK, Ryall RD, Heald RJ. Mesorectal excision for rectal cancer. Lancet 1993;341:457-60.
11. Heald RJ, Moran BJ, Ryall RD, Sexton R, MacFarlane JK. Rectal Cancer: the Basingstoke experience of total mesorectal excision, 1978-1997 Arch Surg 1998;133:894-9.

12. Scheidbach H, Schneider C, Baerlehner E, Konradt J, Koeckerling F. Laparoscopic Colorectal Surgery Study Group. Laparoscopic anterior resection for rectal carcinoma. Results of a registry. Surg Oncol Clin N Am 2001;10:599-609.

13. Anthuber M, Fuerst A, Elser F, Berger R, Jauch KW. Outcome of laparoscopic surgery for rectal cancer in 101 patients. Dis Colon Rectum 2003;46:1047-53.

14. Pilarsky AJ, Rosenthal R, Weiss EG, Wexner SD. Local recurrence and survival after laparoscopic mesorectal excision for rectal adenocarcinoma. Surg Endosc 2002;16:989-95.

15. Yamamoto S, Watanabe M, Hasegawa H, Kitajima. Prospective evaluation of laparoscopic surgery for rectosigmoid and rectal carcinoma. Dis Colon Rectum 2002;45:1648-54.

16. Bretagnol F, Lelong B, Laurent C, et al. The oncological safety of laparoscopic total mesorectal excision with sphincter preservation for rectal carcinoma. Surg Endosc 2005;19:892-6.

17. Zhou ZG, Hu M, Li Y, Lei WZ, Yu YY, Cheng Z, et al. Laparoscopic versus open total mesorectal excision with anal sphincter preservation for low rectal cancer. Surg Endosc 2004;18:1211-5.

18. Lujan J, Valero G, Hernandez Q, Sanchez A, Frutos MD, Parrilla P. Randomized clinical trial comparing laparoscopic and open surgery in patients with rectal cancer. Br J Surg 2009;96:982-9.

19. Guillou PJ, Quirke P, Thorpe H, et al. Short-term endpoints of conventional versus laparoscopic-assisted surgery in patients with colorectal cancer (MRC CLASICC trial): multicentre, randomized controlled trial. Lancet 2005;365:1718-26.

20. Jayne DG, Guillou PJ, Thorpe H, et al. Randomized trial of laparoscopic-assisted resection of colorectal carcinoma: 3-year results of the UK MRC CLASICC Trial Group. J Clin Oncol 2007;25:3061-8.

21. Tekkis PP, Senagore AJ, Delaney CP, Fazio VW. Evaluation of the learning curve in laparoscopic colorectal surgery: comparison of right-sided and left-sided resections. Ann Surg 2005;242:83-91.

22. Anderson C, Uman G, Pigazzi A. Oncologic outcomes of laparoscopic surgery for rectal cancer: A systematic review and meta-analysis of the literature. Eur J Surg Oncol 2008;34:1135-42.

23. Laurent C, Leblanc F, Wutrich P, Scheffler M, Rullier E. Laparoscopic versus open surgery for rectal cancer: long-term oncologic results. Ann Surg 2009;250:54-61.

24. Morino M, Parini U, Giraudo G, Salval M, Brachet Contul R, Garrone C. Laparoscopic total mesorectal excision: a consecutive series of 100 patients. Ann Surg 2003;237:335-42.

25. Tsang WW, Chung CC, Kwok SY, Li MK. Laparoscopic sphincter-preserving total mesorectal excision with colonic J-pouch reconstruction: five-year results. Ann Surg 2006;243:353-8.

26. Leroy J, Jamali F, Forbes L, Smith M, Rubino F, Mutter D, Marescaux J. Laparoscopic total mesorectal excision (TME) for rectal cancer surgery: long-term outcomes. Surg Endosc 2004;18:281-9.

27. Morino M, Allax M, Giraudo G, et al. Laparoscopic versus open surgery for extraperitoneal rectal cancer. Surg Endosc 2005;19:1460-7.

28. Strohlein M, Grutzner K, Jauch K, et al. Comparison of laparoscopic vs open access surgery in patients with rectal cancer: a prospective analysis. Dis Colon Rectum 2008;51:385-91.

29. Lacy A, Garcia-Valdescasa J, Delgado S, et al. Laparoscopy-assisted colectomy versus open colectomy for treatment of non-metastatic colon cancer: a randomised trial. Lancet 2002;359:2224-9.

30. Kapiteijn E, Marijnen CAM, Nagtegaal ID, et al. Preoperative radiotherapy combined with total mesorectal excision for resectable rectal cancer. N Engl J Med 2001;345:638-46.

31. Breukink SO, Pierie JP, Grond AJ, Hoff C, Wiggers T, Meijerink WJ. Laparoscopic versus open total mesorectal excision: a case-control study. Int J Colorectal Dis 2005;20:428-33.

32. Liang JT, Lai HS, Lee PH. Laparoscopic pelvic autonomic nerve-preserving surgery for patients with lower rectal cancer after chemo-radiation therapy. Ann Surg Oncol 2007;14:1285-7.

33. Asoglu O, Matlim T, Karanlik H, et al. Impact of laparoscopic surgery on bladder and sexual function after total mesorectal excision for rectal cancer. Surg Endosc 2009;23:296-303.

34. Jayne DG, Brown JM, Thorpe H, Walker J, Quirke P, Guillou PJ. Bladder and sexual function following resection for rectal cancer in a randomized clinical trial of laparoscopic versus open technique. Br J Surg 2005;92:1124-32.

35. Martling A, Holm T, Rutqvist LE, Johansson H, Moran BJ, Heald RJ, et al. Impact of a surgical training programme on rectal cancer outcomes in Stockholm. Br J Surg 2005;92:225-9.

36. Martling AL, Holm T, Rutqvist LE, Moran BJ, Heald RJ, Cedermark B. Effect of a surgical training programme on outcome of rectal cancer in the County of Stockholm. Stockholm Colorectal Cancer Study Group, Basingstoke Bowel Cancer Research Project. Lancet 2000;356:93-6.

37. Senagore AJ, Stulberg JJ, Byrnes J, et al. A national comparison of laparo-scopic vs. open colectomy using the National Surgical Quality Improvement Project data. Dis Colon Rectum 2009;52(2):183-6.

38. Tan PY, Stephens JH, Rieger NA, et al. Laparoscopically assisted colectomy: a study of risk factors and predictors of open conversion. Surg Endosc 2008;22(7):1708-14.

39. Hemandas AK, Rahman TA, Flashman KG, Skull AJ, Senapati A, O'Leary DP, et al. Laparoscopic Colorectal surgery offers better outcome for high risk cancer patients as compared to open surgery. In Press Annals of Surgery 2010.

40. Pikarsky AJ, Saida Y, Yamagucki T, et al. Is obesity a high-risk factor for laparoscopic colorectal surgery? Surg Endosc 2002;16:855-8.

41. Lee WS, Yun SH, Roh YN, et al. Risk factors and clinical outcome for anastomotic leakage after total mesorectal excision for rectal cancer. World J Surg 2008;32:1124-9.

42. Laurent C, Leblanc F, Gineste C, Saric J, Rullier E. Laparoscopic approach in surgical treatment of rectal cancer. Br J Surg 2007;94:1555-61.

43. Staudacher C, Di PS, Tamburini A, et al. Total mesorectal excision (TME) with laparoscopic approach: 226 consecutive cases. Surg Oncol 2007;16:S113-6.

44. Ng KH, Ng DC, Cheung HY, et al. Laparoscopic resection for rectal cancers: lessons learned from 579 cases. Ann Surg 2009;249:82-6.

45. Brannigan AE, De Buck S, Suetens P, Penninckx F, D'Hoore A. Intracorporeal rectal stapling following laparoscopic total mesorectal excision: overcoming a challenge. Surg Endosc 2006;20:952-5.

46. Brennan DJ, Moynagh M, Brannigan AE, Gleeson F, Rowland M, O'Connell PR. Routine mobilisation of the splenic flexure is not necessary during anterior resection for rectal cancer. Dis Colon Rectum 2007;50:302-7.

47. Weber PA, Merola S, Wasielewski A, Ballantyne GH. Telerobotic assisted laparoscopic right and sigmoid colectomies for benign disease. Dis Colon Rectum 2002;45:1689-94.

48. Munz Y, Moorthy K, Kudchadkar R, et al. Robotic assisted rectopexy. Am J Surg 2004;187:88-92.

49. D'Annibale A, Morpurgo E, Fiscon V. Robotic and laparoscopic surgery for treatment of colorectal diseases. Dis Colon Rectum 2004;47:2162-8.

50. Rockall TA, Darzi A. Robot-assisted laparoscopic colorectal surgery. Surg Clin North Am 2003;83:1463-8.

51. Gutt CN, Oniu T, Mehrabi A, et al. Robot-assisted abdominal surgery. Br J Surg 2004;91:1390-7.

52. Patriti A, Ceccarelli G, Bartoli A, et al. Short- and medium-term outcome of robot-assisted and traditional laparoscopic rectal resection. JSLS 2009;13:176-83.

53. National Cancer Institute. A Phase III Prospective Randomized Trial comparing Laparoscopic-Assisted Resection versus Open resection for rectal cancer. http://clinicaltrials.gov/ct2/show/NCT00726622.

54. Color II Study Group. Color II. A randomized clinical trial comparing laparoscopic and open surgery for rectal cancer. Dan Med Bull 2009;56:89-91.

55. Lelong B, Bege T, Esterni B, et al. Short-term outcome after laparoscopic or open restorative mesorectal excision for rectal cancer: a comparative cohort study. Dis Colon Rectum 2007;50: 76-83.

56. Rezvani M, Franko J, Fassler SA, Harper SG, Nejman JH, Zebley DM. Outcomes in patients treated by laparoscopic resection of rectal carcinoma after neoadjuvant therapy for rectal cancer. JSLS 2007;11:204-7.

57. Tjandra JJ, Chan MK, Yeh CH. Laparoscopic-vs. Hand-assisted ultralow anterior resection: a prospective study. Dis Colon Rectum 2008;51:26-31.

58. Kim SH, Park IJ, Joh YG, Hahn KY. Laparoscopic resection for rectal cancer: a prospective analysis of thirty-month follow-up outcomes in 312 patients. Surg Endosc 2006;20:1197-1202.

59. Lee SI, Kim SH, Wang HM, et al. Local recurrence after laparoscopic resection of T3 rectal cancer without preoperative chemoradiation and a risk group analysis: an Asian collaborative study. J Gastrointest Surg 2008;12: 933-8.

60. Bianchi PP, Rosati R, Bona S, et al. Laparoscopic surgery in rectal cancer: a prospective analysis of patient survival and outcomes. Dis Colon Rectum 2007;50:2047-53.

61. Braga M, Frasson M, Vignali A, Zuliani W, Capretti G, Di Carlo V. Laparoscopic resection in rectal cancer patients: outcome and cost-benefit analysis. Dis Colon Rectum 2007;50:464-71.

CHAPTER ELEVEN

Therapeutic Endoscopy in Gastrointestinal Cancers

Sunil Kumar, Arunima Verma

INTRODUCTION

Endoscopy has a significant role to play in the medical and surgical management of gastrointestinal cancers both in localized and advanced conditions. With the emergence of natural orifice transluminal endoscopic surgery (NOTES), there is renewed interest among surgeons for endoscopy. The diagnostic potentials of endoscopy are already established and with technological advancements and technique refinements, therapeutic endoscopy is making a mark in management—both palliative and curative—in gastrointestinal malignancies.

THERAPEUTIC ENDOSCOPIC MODALITIES FOR GASTROINTESTINAL (GI) CANCERS

Endoscopic stenting, photodynamic treatment, laser treatment, argon plasma coagulation, and endoscopic mucosal resection and endoscopic submucosal dissection are all used in various malignant conditions of the gastrointestinal tract.

Endoscopic Stenting

A stent is a device inserted into the body to treat an obstruction due to benign or malignant cause. In the gastrointestinal system stents are used in the esophagus, stomach, pancreas, bile ducts and the rectum and colon. The stents are usually made of medical grade plastic or metals and are open at both ends to facilitate the passage of food, liquids or body fluids. There are differences in the type of stent and technique used, depending on the area to be stented.

Stent placement may cause complications, of which bleeding, perforation, stent migration and tumor ingrowth and overgrowth are well known. Different types are used, to increase clinical success and reduce complication rates. Biodegradeable stents for benign disease and radioactive or drug-eluting stents for malignant disease are in the process of development.

Photodynamic Therapy

Photodynamic therapy (PDT) is an ablative treatment for rapidly proliferating tissues, including dysplastic and malignant lesions.[1] The principle underlying PDT is that a photosensitizer is exposed to intense white or specific wavelength light and this leads to a photochemical reaction, which produces singlet oxygen radicals. This singlet oxygen and other reactive chemical radicals cause local non-thermal cellular damage, vascular thrombosis and necrosis, which evolve over hours to several days. Cellular localization and depth of injury depend upon the sensitizing agent, interval between dosing and light stimulation, and the light dosimetry and wavelength. The endoscopic photodynamic therapy device consists of a multitude of low wattage diodes at the distal end of the endoscope, a scattering glass, cooling channel, external cooling unit, an inflatable balloon with a reflective surface and a tube connected to an external pump for the delivery and removal of photosensitizer. The photosensitizing agent may have a tropism for faster growing malignant cells or may be simply retained in these tissues owing to poor lymphatic drainage.[8]

The photosensitizing agents are based upon modifications of porphyrin, chlorine and chlorophyll whose macromolecular nature causes preferential localization within and delayed clearance from the neoplastic tissue, leading to a degree of selective treatment when tissue is stimulated with light. Porfimer sodium and 5-aminolevulinic acid (5-ALA) are the photosensitizing agents currently in use.[2,3] Both agents absorb light preferentially in the range 630 to 635 nm. Longer wavelengths of light penetrate tissue more effectively than shorter wavelength.

The usual treatment regime used in gastrointestinal malignancy is 2 mg/kg IV Porfimer sodium for all GI malignancies with a light dose varying from 150 to 300 J/cm. Most tissues are treated with a single dose of photosensitizer, followed by one application of 630 nm laser light 40 to 50 hours after infusion of the photosensitizing drug. Subsequent full courses of PDT up to 3 total can be used after 1 to 3 months or more.

Indications of PDT in GI malignancies are for
1. Palliative treatment of patients with completely or partially obstructing esophageal cancer.
2. Treatment of superficial gastric carcinoma.[1]
3. Palliative treatment for non-resectable cholangiocarcinoma. [4]
4. Extensive FAP associated adenomas of the duodenum or colorectum.[5]

PDT is a relatively expensive treatment modality and side effects like photosensitizer induced skin injury and luminal stricture of the ablation site may occur. Patients should wear protective clothing and avoid sunlight because most sunscreen block out only ultraviolet (UV) light but not the damaging infrared light.[6,7]

Key Point

- Photodynamic therapy is based on the principle of photochemical reaction between photosensitizer agent and laser light, which releases singlet oxygen radicals. These cause cell necrosis and death.

Argon Plasma Coagulation

The argon plasma coagulation (APC) has multiple applications in the GI tract. APC is a type of monopolar coagulation based mainly on the effects of high-frequency electrical current flowing through a conductive and ionized argon medium.[8] It is less expensive compared to the Nd:YAG laser. Because of its inherent properties, it is difficult to treat an area that has been previously desiccated, thus, reducing the risk of perforation. This technique destroys tissue to a depth of 1 to 3 mm.[9] It is useful in eradication of flat neoplastic tissue that is not amenable to removal by snare polypectomy and also in recanalization in luminal malignant obstruction like that in the esophagus. Since this technique destroys tissue without allowing retrieval for histologic evaluation, it is recommended for use only for residual sessile tissue and for palliation in proved malignant obstruction.

Key Point

- Argon plasma coagulation is useful in eradication of flat neoplastic tissue and recanalization in luminal malignant obstruction.

Endoscopic Mucosal Resection (EMR) and Endoscopic Submucosal Dissection (ESD)

EMR and ESD are used for treatment of early malignant lesions limited to mucosa in the esophagus, stomach and colon. EMR serves both diagnostic and therapeutic role. A lesion can be entirely resected by EMR and when histopathological assessment proves the resected margin to be clear, it is curative.[13] Several EMR techniques are currently used in clinical practice[15] and innovations continue. The techniques in use are:
1. The "inject and cut" technique.
2. The "simple snare" resection technique.
3. The "cap" technique.
4. The ligation technique. The other innovations in technique include submucosal endoscopy but are in experimental phase.[16]

149

The gold standard for endoscopic mucosal resection is a one-piece resection of the lesion as it not only allows an accurate histological assessment, but also reduces the risk of recurrence.[17,18] The limitation of EMR is that only lesions with diameter 20 mm or less can be resected enbloc. Moreover, ulcerated lesions often have fibrosis, which can lead to failure to lift the lesion.[13] Larger lesions have been resected by using the piecemeal technique but there are chances of recurrence as there would be small neoplastic residues due to inefficient overlapping of resection areas.[19] Complications of EMR include bleeding and perforation.

To overcome the limitations of EMR, a new technique, endoscopic submucosal dissection (ESD) was developed, which was initially used for early neoplastic resections in the stomach but is now used at various other sites like esophagus and colon. In ESD, the submucosal layer underneath the carcinoma is dissected to obtain a larger mucosal specimen, with the neoplasm resected en bloc. Complications of bleeding and perforation are more frequent with ESD compared to EMR and it needs more procedure time.

Key Point

- EMR and ESD are used for the treatment of early malignant lesions limited to the mucosa in the esophagus, stomach and colon.

THERAPEUTIC ENDOSCOPY FOR ESOPHAGEAL CANCER

Esophageal cancer is the seventh most common cause of cancer death.[10] Surgical resection[12] is the only hope for cure, but despite the advances in therapy, more than 50% of them are incurable at the time of presentation. Even with resection, prognosis is poor, with 40% of patients dying in the first year of surgery and 5-year survival rates of 27%.[13] Endoscopic ultrasound (EUS) has become the standard practice for staging esophageal cancer based on the diagnostic accuracy of the test. EUS also identifies patients who would benefit from endoscopic modalities like EMR.[31] Therapeutic endoscopy has both curative and palliative roles in esophageal cancer.

Endoscopic screening programs have made possible the diagnosis of early esophageal cancers, which include high grade intraepithelial neoplasia (HGIN) and esophageal cancer confined to the mucosa only, for which curative endoscopic options like ablative therapies and EMR can be used.[11,13]

CURATIVE ENDOSCOPIC THERAPIES

Ablative Therapy

The various ablative techniques used are PDT, APC and multipolar electrocoagulation. Ultrasonic energy and liquid nitrogen are also used for the destruction of Barrett's esophagus. These therapies may be associated with complications like stricture, deep thermal injury and perforation. The recent addition to this group is endoscopic radio-frequency ablation (RFA) either circumferential or focal. This has shown promising results in HGIN and Barrett's esophagus, but more studies and long-term follow-up are needed to establish its role.

The end result of successful ablative therapy is the complete eradication of carcinomatous, dysplastic or sometimes even the metaplastic (Barrett's esophagus) tissue. The destroyed tissue targeted by ablative therapy re-epithelializes with squamous mucosa.[14]

Endoscopic Mucosal Resection

Various studies have proved EMR to be a safe and effective technique for early squamous cell cancer of the esophagus. The complete response rate from 10 series varied between 92 and 100%. Recurrent/metachronous lesions were seen in 0 to 26%.[13] Besides bleeding and perforation, the other main complication of EMR in esophagus is stricture formation. ESD has also been used in early esophageal cancer but more studies are needed to establish its use in esophageal cancer.

PALLIATIVE ENDOSCOPIC THERAPY

Palliation of esophageal carcinoma mainly consists of the symptomatic relief of dyshagia.[20] This is evaluated by the quality of swallowing assessed with the dysphagia score, which ranges from 0 for normal swallowing to 4 for complete dysphagia as described by Mellow and Pinkas[21] (Table 11.1).

Surgery is not used commonly for palliative treatment because of the associated high morbidity and mortality rates. Palliative options are chemotherapy, radiotherapy and endoscopic palliation techniques. The endoscopic palliation techniques for advanced esophageal cancer are varied, but most frequently used is stent placement.[13] The other palliative options are—alcohol injection, laser therapy, APC, PDT and brachy-therapy.

TABLE 11.1

Dysphagia score as described by Mellow and Pinkas [21]

Score	Quality of swallowing
0	Ability to eat normal diet
1	Ability to eat some solid food
2	Ability to eat semisolids only
3	Ability to swallow liquids only
4	Complete dysphagia

Alcohol Injection

Direct injection of pure ethanol into malignant tissue is a simple and cheap technique used for recanalization of the esophagus.[8] Alcohol is injected under endoscopic visualization and it causes tumor ulceration and necrosis leading to relief of malignant dysphagia. 0.25 ml alcohol is injected per site with a total of 7 to 10 ml per session. Therapy is repeated weekly until the desired effect is achieved, which in most cases takes 2 to 3 sessions. Thereafter, the procedure is repeated on a monthly basis to maintain luminal patency.[21] Significant relief of dysphagia has been seen in two uncontrolled studies.[22,23] Overzealous injection should be avoided to reduce the risk of perforation.

Laser Therapy

Laser therapy involves the use of laser light to coagulate tissue under endoscopic guidance; most commonly used is the neodymium-doped yttrium aluminium garnet (Nd:YAG) laser.[8] Laser therapy is useful for tumor debulking, luminal expansion and control of bleeding. It cannot be used for infiltrative scirrhous type tumor or in the presence of fistulas.[21] It is an effective modality in the treatment of malignant esophageal obstruction with a success rate of 75 to 91%.[24,25] Laser therapy needs repeated sessions at regular intervals of approximately four weeks and earlier in some cases when rapid disease progression makes the dysphagia free interval shorter.[20] Complications include perforation, bleeding and formation of tracheoesophageal fistulas.

The cost incurred by laser therapy is almost the same as stenting, which needs less intervention. Hence, laser therapy is usually reserved for proximal esophageal lesions where stenting is not feasible,[8] for tumor debulking prior to stent placement or for treatment of tumor ingrowth of a stent.[21]

Esophageal Stenting

Using a stent to relieve the obstruction within the esophagus was proposed as early as the mid 19th century. Nowadays, there are various types of stent available with various features aimed at preventing complications. The first generation stents are the rigid plastic stents, which are obsolete now as many studies have proved the superiority of self expanding metal stents (SEMS).[26-30] These SEMS represent the second generation and are made up of nitinol, stainless steel or other alloys. They can be uncovered or covered with a polyurethane or silicone liner. Further modification is the addition of an antireflux valve. The commercially available esophageal stents include the Ultraflex (Microinvasive, Boston Scientific, USA), the Z-stent (Wilson-Cook Medical, USA), the Bonastent (standard Sci-Tech,

Korea), the Choo stent (MI Tech, Korea) and the Niti-S –Stent (Taewoong Medical, Korea). Third generation stents are self-expanding plastic stents (SEPS), which have a polyurethane mesh with a silicone coating, commercially available as polyflex stent (Boston Scientific, Natick, Massachusetts). The fourth generation consists of bioabsorbable stents made of poly- L- lactide, which prevent the complications of stent removal and have been proposed for airways and esophagus.[32]

The choice of stent in an individual is influenced by a variety of factors including tumor length and position, presence of a fistula, potential airway compromise and personal preference of the individual inserting the stent. The diameter and length of the stricture is determined by fluoroscopy and endoscopy. The chosen stent should have a length at least 3 to 4 cm longer than the obstruction to allow an adequate margin of stent on either side of the obstruction.

It has been convincingly shown that the partially or fully covered metal stents give better long-term palliation of malignant dysphagia than uncovered stents.[33] SEPS has the advantage of being removable even after several months while SEMS are permanent.[8]

Procedure related complications after stent placement occur in 5 to 10% patients and mainly consist of perforation, aspiration pneumonia, fever, hemorrhage and severe pain. Delayed complications with recurrent dysphagia are reported in 30 to 40% patients and include hemorrhage, fistula formation, stent migration, tissue in growth or overgrowth and food-bolus obstruction.

Tumors close to the upper esophageal sphincter (UES) are traditionally the most difficult to manage and stents at this location have additional complications like patient intolerance due to pain and globus sensation, besides the increased risks of perforation, aspiration pneumonia, tracheo-esophageal fistula formation and proximal migration.[35] Newly designed stents with shorter length of upper flange (7 mm) and ultraflex have been used with success in this situation and optimal results are achieved with expertise. Now stents can be used for palliation of malignant stricture close to the UES.[35]

Tumors of the distal esophagus and gastric cardia are associated with specific problem like gastroesophageal reflux and stent migration as the distal part of the stent projects freely into the fundus of the stomach and cannot fix itself to the wall. Here, stents with antireflux valves like Dua Z stent, Choo stent and Bonastent with "Shim's modification" are used.[34]

Innovations continue and combination of brachytherapy with stent is possible by using an esophageal stent loaded with iodine-125 seeds. It has been reported that this stent provided slightly longer relief of dysphagia and extended survival.[36]

Stenting is the most commonly used technique for endoscopic palliation and is safe and effective for esophageal cancer at any site.

Brachytherapy

Intraluminal brachytherapy with cobalt 60 and iridium 192 has been widely used in esophageal cancer, with the achievement of palliation and few complications.[37-39] In a study conducted by Homs et al, it was seen that single-dose brachytherapy gave better long-term relief of dysphagia with fewer complications than metal stent placement.[38] Also, brachytherapy is recommended for patients with life expectancy longer than 3 months as it gives better dysphagia-adjusted survival compared to stents, which are recommended for patients with life-expectancy less than 3 months. Complications include procedure-related complications and late complications like fistula formation and bleeding.

Others

For palliation of esophageal luminal obstruction PDT and APC have been used. Studies have shown recanalization rates with APC between 86 and 89%.[40,41] APC sessions at 3 to 4 weeks interval is needed to maintain luminal patency and esophageal perforation may occur in 1 to 1.8% of cases.[8]

Key Points

- Therapeutic endoscopy has both curative and palliative roles in carcinoma of the esophagus.
- Curative options are ablative therapies and endoscopic mucosal resection (EMR).
- Endoscopic palliation of esophageal carcinoma mainly consists of the symptomatic relief of dysphagia.
- Stent is the most commonly used endoscopic palliation technique and is safe and effective for esophageal cancer at any site.
- Other endoscopic palliation techniques for esophageal cancer are alcohol injection, laser therapy, APC, PDT and brachytherapy.

THERAPEUTIC ENDOSCOPY FOR GASTRODUODENAL MALIGNANCY

Gastric cancer is the second most common fatal malignancy worldwide. Endoscopic surveillance has made possible the detection of early gastric cancer (EGC) in which the adenocarcinoma invasion is limited to the lamina propria or submucosa, independent of lymph node status. This group represents about 50 and 20% of the newly diagnosed gastric cancers in Japan and in the West, respectively.[67-71] Also gastric polyps are found to be present in less than 1% of the general population; 90% of these are hyperplastic polyps, which are small and rarely more than 1.5 cm. Rate of malignant transformation in these is low but increases with increasing size in polyps larger than 1 cm. Endoscopic polypectomy followed by endoscopic screening is recommended for these polyps.

Tumor Ablation in the Stomach

EMR for EGC is a curative technique that avoids surgery and its potential complications. With EUS, the exact depth can be assessed in approximately 80% cases of gastric cancer. EMR can be used for EGC lesions smaller than 2 to 3 cm as these have only 3.5% chance of lymph node involvement. Lesions more than 4.5 cm have a more than 50% chance of spread into submucosa with positive lymph nodes. Hence, lesions amenable to curative resection by EMR are those limited to mucosa with negative lymph nodes confirmed by EUS; size less than 2 cm for slightly elevated lesions and size less than 1 cm for slightly depressed lesions without ulcer scar; no evidence of multiple gastric cancer or simultaneous abdominal malignancy and histologically cancer of intestinal type. Sites difficult to access by EMR are the lesser curvature, posterior wall of the gastric body, the cardia and lesser curvature of the antrum. Overall recurrence rate is about 10% (0% when resection is complete and 35% when resection is incomplete.[72] Tumor free margin is important as there is a recurrence of 37 to 50% for tumor positive margins as reported in various series.[73-75] The subsequent need for surgery is decided upon the microscopic evaluation of the specimen.[76]

ESD can achieve large en bloc resection through a standard single channel gastroscope with lower recurrence than in EMR. One study showed 92.8% rate of curative treatment with ESD for gastric epithelial tumors.[77]

PDT can be used in patients who refuse surgery or are unfit for surgery due to comorbidities, but the use of PDT for palliation in gastric cancer needs further study.

ENDOSCOPIC STENTING OF THE STOMACH AND DUODENUM

The other area suitable for endoscopic intervention in gastroduodenal malignancies is malignant gastric outlet obstruction (GOO). Causes of malignant GOO are mostly advanced upper gastrointestinal malignancies like those of pancreas, ampulla, gastric or cholangiocarcinoma or due to metastatic tumors to stomach or duodenum. Endoscopic techniques used for palliation of GOO are enteral stents, laser therapy and APC. Enteral stents are mostly self-expanding metal stents similar to the esophageal, biliary and colonic stents and are metal mesh stent put across malignant gastroduodenal strictures or obstruction with an endoscope under fluoroscopic guidance. They are permanent devices not intended to be removed after placement. Complications are the same as for SEMS at other locations. APC can be used for endoscopic fenestration of these duodenal stents to facilitate endoscopic retrograde cholangiopancreatography (ERCP) if need be.[78]

Key Points

- EMR for EGC is a curative technique and avoids surgery and its potential complications.
- Enteral stents, laser therapy and APC are used for palliation of GOO.

THERAPEUTIC ENDOSCOPY IN PANCREATICOBILIARY MALIGNANCIES

Malignancies of the biliary and pancreatic system are not uncommon and cause malignant biliary obstruction. Metastatic lesions to the head of pancreas or porta hepatis also may cause biliary obstruction. The location of the obstruction within the biliary tree is important with regards to the palliative approach within each discipline and is generally divided into non-hilar and hilar biliary obstruction.[44]

Distal or Non-Hilar Biliary Obstruction

The most common cancer causing distal biliary malignant obstruction is pancreatic cancer[42] followed by gallbladder cancer, malignant lymphadenopathy, cholangiocarcinoma and carcinoma of ampulla of vater. The overall prognosis of these malignancies is dismal and the majority of patients are diagnosed with unresectable disease with a median survival of 3-5 months.[43] Only 10 to 20% of cases are amenable to curative resection. Moreover, as the median age of diagnosis of pancreaticobiliary malignancies is approximately 70 years, many of these patients are judged unfit for surgery due to advanced age and existing comorbidities. Thus, most of the patients need palliative treatment in the form of surgical bypass or biliary stenting—percutaneous or endoscopic.

Endoscopic approaches are considered first line treatment of palliation in these inoperable malignancies, causing distal biliary obstruction.[45] The conditions for which palliation is needed are cholestasis, pain and gastrointestinal obstruction. ERCP biliary stenting is effective for the relief of cholestasis leading to cholangitis and pruritus. The biliary stents are of two types—plastic stents and self-expanding metal stents (covered and uncovered).

Biliary Plastic Stents

Plastic stents were first introduced in 1979 by Soehendra and Reynders-Frederix[46] and are made up of polyethylene polymer or Teflon. They are inexpensive and removable, but their small lumen renders them susceptible to loss of patency within an average of 3 to 4 months because of formation of adherent bacterial biofilm and accumulation of biliary sludge.[47] The biofilm consists of cellular debris and microcolonies of bacteria in a matrix of extracellular anionic fibrillar material.[48] Larger stents of 10 or 11.5 F diameter remain patent two to three times longer than

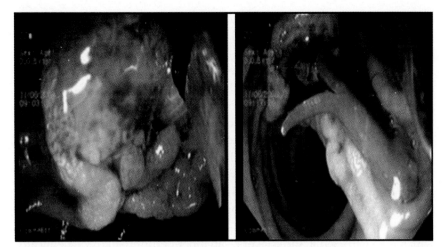

Fig. 11.1: ERCP stenting of ampullary carcinoma. A 62-year-old man with obstructive jaundice with S. bilirubin of 24 mg% underwent ERCP and periampullary growth found, which was biopsied and stented with 8.5 F plastic stent and the patient later underwent Whipple's operation.

7 or 8 F diameter stent but stent diameter is limited by the diameter of the accessory channel of the endoscope.[49] Clinical evidence is that 11.5 F stents have not shown prolonged patency compared to 10 F stent. Hence, 10 F tents are usually preferred.[50-52] Innovations in the design of plastic stent continue to eliminate obstruction from biofilm or sludge formation and to this end a "winged" stent has been designed, which facilitates the flow of bile around the stent with potential to prolong the biliary drainage. Prospective comparative trials are needed to define the role of this novel stent design.[45]

For the deployment of a large diameter plastic stent, some endoscopists prefer to do an endoscopic sphincterotomy (ES), but a prospective study showed that this is not necessary for the placement of 10 F plastic stent in patients with malignant common bile duct (CBD) obstruction, rather the complications were higher in the group where ES was used.[53]

The use of a plastic stent is recommended in patients with poor prognosis with life-expectancy less than 5-6 months (Fig. 11.1).[53]

Biliary Self-Expanding Metal Stents

Self-expanding metal stents (SEMS) were introduced at the end of the 1980s to overcome the disadvantages of plastic stents. SEMS have the combined advantage of a small predeployment delivery system with a large postdeployment stent diameter and also have longer duration of patency and less stent failure. The early uncovered SEMS were susceptible to obstruction due to tumor ingrowth, tumor overgrowth or tissue hyperplasia.[44] To protect against tumor ingrowth, covered SEMS were developed in 1990s. Currently, several types of biliary SEMS are available, varying in shape, design and metal alloy. For example, wallstent (Boston scientific), the Zilver stent (Wilson-Cook Medical), Luminex (Bard) and Ultraflex diamond (Boston Scientific). A prospective randomized study of "covered" versus "uncovered" diamond stent for the management of distal malignant biliary obstruction concluded that covered diamond stents were significantly superior to uncovered diamond stents in terms of patency.[49] In this study, stent obstruction occurred in 14% of covered stents and 38% uncovered stents. The complications specific to covered stents are acute cholecystitis and pancreatitis. Also, stent migration is more common with covered stents, which may also become occluded by adherence of bacteria to the membrane coating.[45]

A recent development in stents is the advent of a double-layered stent, which is constructed in three layers—an inner perfluoroalkoxy (chemically smoothed Teflon) layer, an outer stiff polyamide elastomer and a middle stainless steel mesh that holds the inner and outer layers together. The cost of this stent is similar to polyethylene stent and it is reported to have a longer patency in a randomized trial,[54] but further studies are needed to confirm the findings.

Next in line are the drug-eluting biliary SEMS in which stents covered with chemotherapeutic agent, like paclitaxel, are used to retard tumor growth. This has been studied in animal models but clinical trials are awaited to further establish their safety and efficacy.[45] Considering the cost of SEMS, they should be used in patients expected to survive longer than six months.

Pancreatic Stenting

Pain related to pancreatic duct obstruction occurs in approximately 15% of patients with advanced pancreatic cancer. Endoscopic palliation in the form of ERCP pancreatic stenting in subjects with a dilated main pancreatic duct above the stricture, confirmed by computed tomography (CT) or magnetic resonance cholangiopancreatography (MRCP), effectively makes 50 to 60% subjects symptom free and 20 to 25% have significantly reduced amounts of analgesic consumption. The exact timing of stent exchange has not been studied so far.[45] Endoscopic pancreatic stenting should be considered in selected patients for obstructive pain not responding to analgesics.

Hilar Biliary Obstruction

Hilar obstructions are usually caused by cholangiocarcinoma, metastatic disease, central intrahepatic masses and gallbladder cancer. Compared to distal biliary obstruction, the clinical success rates of palliation is less for hilar obstruction. Prosthetic palliation of patients with malignant hilar stenoses poses difficulties, especially in advanced lesions (type II or higher). The risk of cholangitis after contrast injection into the biliary tree in cases where incomplete drainage is achieved is well known. Retention of contrast and subsequent segmental cholangitis is a risk associated with endoscopic attempts to treat advanced hilar lesions. Percutaneous transhepatic cholangiography (PTC) may permit percutaneous drainage targeted to the desired duct system and is usually preferred for hilar obstruction. Hilar obstruction may be treated with ERCP stenting and PDT if PTC is not available.

It is not firmly established that metal stents offer superior prolongation of palliation compared with plastic stents, as seen in distal strictures. Uncovered metal stents are better for hilar obstruction as stent migration is less compared to cover SEMS.

Other endoscopic palliations used for hilar cholangiocarcinoma are PDT and also in trial is the cyberknife stereotactic radiotherapy in which radiographic markers (fiducials) are implanted at the tumor site as reference points by endoscopic ultrasound (EUS) guided placement (instead of surgical or percutaneous placement under USG or CT guidance) and radiation beams are targeted at them.

Further endoscopic palliation in biliary obstruction includes endoscopic management of stent occlusion. In a retrospective analysis it was seen that the use of SEMS as initial intervention in patients with occluded SEMS provides longer patency and survival and can decrease the number of subsequent ERCPs by 50% compared to plastic stents.[55] The use of APC and laser therapy have also been reported but this needs further study.

Key Points

- The location of biliary obstruction is important with regards to palliative approach.
- Endoscopic palliation is indicated for cholangitis and pruritus due to cholestasis and is provided by ERCP stenting.
- The use of plastic stents is nowadays recommended in patients with poor prognosis with life expectancy less than 5–6 months.
- SEMS should be used in patients expected to survive longer than six months.
- Endoscopic pancreatic stenting should be considered for obstructive pain not responding to analgesics in selected patients.
- Hilar obstruction may be treated with ERCP stenting and PDT if PTC is not available.

THERAPEUTIC ENDOSCOPY IN COLORECTAL MALIGNANCY

Colorectal cancer is the third most commonly diagnosed cancer and second leading cause of death for both men and women in the United **159**

States[56] where it is predicted to develop in 106,000 and 40,000 individuals, respectively.[8] Throughout the world, colorectal adenomas have been found in 0.8-5.2% of patients undergoing colonoscopies for different indications.[57] The risk of high grade dysplasia and cancer increases with the size of the lesion, hence they should be removed.

Endoscopic therapies are used for prevention of malignant transformation by endoscopic removal of polyps, for palliation of malignant bowel obstruction by various endoscopic techniques and even for cure of early lesions limited to mucosa, by EMR and ESD.

Endoscopic Treatment of Colorectal Lesions

Colonoscopic Polypectomy

Colonoscopic polypectomy is the most effective visceral cancer prevention tool in clinical medicine[58] but ineffective polypectomy leads to colorectal cancer. With the availability of advanced technology like optical enhancement techniques, there is improved exposure of colonic mucosa, the detection of flat lesions and the determination of histology in real time. Generally, all adenomas or potential adenomas should be removed during colonoscopy. All hyperplastic polyps in the proximal colon should be removed. Small distal colon hyperplastic polyps, mucosal polyps and lymphoid hyperplasia, inflammatory polyps and true filiform pseudo-polyps in inflammatory bowel disease (IBD) need not be removed during colonoscopy.

There is no universally accepted single technique for polypectomy despite the need to have a best approach for it as most of the colonic perforations are related to polypectomy.[59] The various methods used for removal of small polyps are cold forceps, hot forceps, hot snare, cold snare and combined methods (Fig. 11.2). Large pedunculated polyps are most common in the sigmoid colon and are removed by polypectomy snare. Various techniques are used to handle the bleeding from the stalk, like injection of epinephrine, application of multipolar electrocautery, detachable snares, clips, endoloops or rubber bands. Piecemeal removal is also used for large-sized polyps. Macroscopic and microscopic clearance of adenomatous tissue at 3- to 6-month follow-up after polypectomy of large adenomas is an excellent predictor of successful eradication.[60]

Large sessile and flat polyps represent a major technical challenge to conventional snare resection. Sessile lesions in sigmoid occupying more than 30% circumference are difficult to remove endoscopically and so are polyps in the cecum, polyps extending into the ileocecal valve orifice or polyps overlying the appendiceal orifice. By contrast, sessile polyps in the rectum, transverse colon or ascending colon that occupy 50 to 60% circumference can be resected endoscopically. Conventional snare

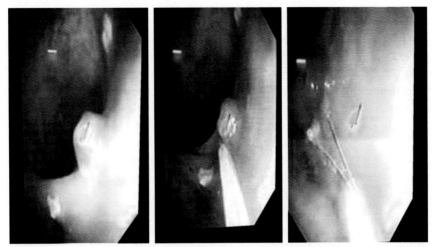

Fig. 11.2: Colonoscopic polypectomy by snare. A 55-year-old man presented with recurrent bleeding per rectum and a sessile polyp was seen in the sigmoid colon, which was resected by snare and sent for biopsy. The histological diagnosis was an adenocarcinoma and the patient was later subjected to left hemicolectomy.

resection is not adequate for large sessile and flat polyps. APC may be used to destroy remnant tissue after resection. EMR has been shown to be useful in resection of large sessile and flat colorectal lesions.

Endoscopic Mucosal Resection (EMR)

In the colon, EMR is indicated for carpet like adenomatous polyps or for moderately well-differentiated or well-differentiated adenocarcinoma confined to the mucosa or extending into the superficial submucosa but with specific surface morphology. EMR is indicated for sessile, flat elevated and lateral spreading tumors, not greater than 2.5 cm in diameter or flat adenomatous lesions or mixed lesions less than 10 mm in diameter.[60] EMR is a safe and effective alternative to surgery for superficial resection in selected patients.

For EMR, the first step is lifting the lesion with injection of fluid, usually saline or sodium hyaluronate and hypertonic dextrose with epinephrine. En bloc removal is possible in small lesions (< 2 cm) and piecemeal removal in larger lesions. The two major techniques used are non-suction (lift-and-cut) and suction (suck-and-cut). Various modifications of these two basic techniques are used. Predictors of difficult EMR and potential need for surgery include large tumors, sessile or flat/ depressed morphology and submucosal invasion. A meta-analysis showed that success rate for en bloc margin free resection is not high but improves with experience.[61] Improvements in technique and equipment are also needed.

Endoscopic Submucosal Dissection (ESD)

With larger colorectal lesions and superficial submucosal invasion, endoscopic submucosal dissection (ESD) has been the area of interest. ESD permits en bloc resection of lesions larger than 5 cm in diameter but is technically difficult, more time consuming and associated with higher rates of bleeding and perforation compared to EMR. The initial technique is like in EMR, i.e. lifting the lesion with injection of a viscous submucosal fluid cushion, such as glycerin, hyaluronon or lubricant jelly, which needs to be repeated from time-to-time to prevent perforation, as the colonic wall is thin and the submucosal fluid leaks during the procedure. Thereafter an electrosurgical knife is used for the submucosal dissection. In one series of 200 colonic neoplasms in 18 patients, with lesions, including adenomas, superficial carcinomas and invasive carcinomas, 91.5% lesions were treated with en bloc resection of which 70.5% had tumor free margin.[62] Further improvements, such as magnetic anchor-guided ESD are in development and more technical advancements may make it possible to use these techniques in the areas inaccessible to endoscopic therapy at present.

Endoscopic Palliation for Malignant Large Bowel Obstruction

Patients with advanced colorectal cancer can present with symptoms of chronic constipation or acute obstruction. There is a need for decompression and clinical stabilization before surgery in these patients for which endoscopic techniques are used nowadays.

Colonic Decompression Tubes

Colonic decompression tubes are inexpensive and widely available and can be implanted with or without endoscopic visualization in patients with residual colonic lumen, or over a guidewire in those with complete obstruction. Large bore colorectal decompression tubes are available, which allow preoperative bowel preparation so that a one-staged surgical procedure is possible.[63]

Self-expanding Metal Stents

Dedicated or specific colorectal stents are available like Enteral Wallstent, Colonic Z-stent (Wilson–Cook Medical Inc.) and Nitinol wire colonic stent (Ultraflex Precision Colonic). The use of fluoroscopy is recommended for deployment of any colonic stent.[8] In one series, the technical success rate was 92% and clinical success rate was 78.8% for colonic SEMS.[64] Colonic stents have not been shown to prolong life.[65,66] Complications of colonic SEMS include improper placement, migration, perforation and bleeding and these occur during or immediately after stent deployment. Tumor ingrowth and tumor overgrowth are late complications occurring days to months after stent placement. Despite the drawbacks of failures, complications and mortality, initial stent insertion compares favorably with emergency surgery either in the setting of a bridge to elective operation or as definitive palliation.

Laser Therapy

As at any other obstructed luminal, laser therapy with Nd:YAG laser can recanalize the obstructed lumen. It cannot be used in the cases of acute obstruction or extrinsic compression by genitourinary cancers or gynecological cancer where SEMS can be used. It relieves obstruction in 75 to 80% patients but requires multiple treatments to maintain patency. Complications are as for laser therapy at other sites like perforation, bleeding, postprocedure pain and formation of fistulas or abscesses.

Argon Plasma Coagulation (APC)

APC may be used for patients with malignant obstruction or to control bleeding from colorectal cancer but data is limited.

Key Points

- Endoscopy is used for surveillance, prevention of premalignant lesions turning into malignant, palliation of malignant bowel obstruction and curative resection in colorectal malignancy.
- Endoscopic treatment of colorectal malignant polyps and adenomas includes polypectomy, EMR and ESD.
- Endoscopic palliation for malignant large bowel obstruction can be achieved by colonic decompression tubes, self-expanding metal stents, laser therapy and APC.

REFERENCES

1. Photodynamic therapy for gastrointestinal disease. Gastrointestinal Endoscopy, 2006;63(7):927-32.
2. Photofirin (Axcan Scandipharm). PDR. net Available at : http://www. pdr. net/druginformation/Document search. aspx?documentid=04250800 anddrugname=Photofrin%20 for % 20 Injection. Accessed May 12, 2006.
3. Messmann H. 5-Aminolevulinic acid-induced protopoirphyrin IX for the detection of gastrointestinal dysplasia. Gastrointestinal Endosc Clin of N Am 2000;10:497-512.
4. Ortner MA, Liebetruth J, Schreiber S, et al. Photodynamic therapy of nonresectable cholangiocarcinoma. Gastroenterology 1998;114:536-42.
5. Mlkvy P, Messmann H, Debinski H, et al. Photodynamic therapy for polyps in familial adenomatous polyposis: a pilot study. Eur J Cancer 1995;31A: 1160-5.

6. Marcon NE. Photodynamic therapy and cancer of the esophagus. Semin Onclo 1994;21 (Suppl 15):20-3.

7. Saidi RF, Marcon NE. Nonthermal ablation of malignant esophageal strictures L: photodynamic therapy, endoscopic intraluminal injections, and novel modalities. Gastrointest Endosc Clin N Am 1998;8:465-91.

8. Douglas G Adler, Shehzad N Merawat. Endoscopic approaches for palliation of luminal Gastrointestinal obstruction. Gastroenterol Clin N Am 2006;35:65-82.

9. Chang Kyun Lee, Suck-HO Lee, Ji-Young Park, Tae Hoon Lee, II-Kwun Chung, Sang-Heum Park, Hong-Soo Kim, et al. Prophylactic Argon Plasma Coagulation ablation does not decrease delayed postpolypectomy bleeding. Gastrointest. Endoscopy 2009;70(2):353-61.

10. Jemal A, Murray T, Samuels A, et al. Cancer statistics 2003, CA Cancer J Clin 2003;53:5-26.

11. Hulscher JB, van Sandick JW, de Boer AG, et al. Extended transthoracic compared with limited transhiatal resection for adenocarcinoma of the esophagus. N Engl J Med 2002;21:1662-9.

12. Muller JM, Erasm H, Stelzner M, et al. Surgical therapy of esophageal cancer. Br J Surg 1990;77:845-57.

13. Peter D Siersema. Esophageal cancer. Gastroenterol Clin N Am 2008;37:943-64.

14. Jennifer R Scudiere, Elizabeth A Montgomery. New treatments, New Challenges: pathology's perspective on esophageal carcinoma. Gastroenterol Clin N Am 2009;38:121-33.

15. Soetikno R, Kaltenbach T, Yeh R, et al. Endoscopic mucosal resection for early cancers of the upper gastrointestinal tract. J Clin Oncol 2005;23:4490-8.

16. Stefan von Delius, Hubertus Feusner, Julia Henke, Armin Schneider Regina Hollweck, Thomas Rösch, et al. Submucosal endoscopy: a novel approach to en bloc endoscopic mucosal resection. Gastrointestinal Endoscopy, 2007; 66(4):753-6.

17. Matsushita M, Hajiro K, Okazaki K, et al. Endoscopic mucosal resection of gastric tumors located in the lesser curvature of upper third of the stomach. Gastrointest Endosc 1997;45:512-5.

18. Okhuwa M, Hosokawa K, Boku N, et al. New endoscopic treatment for intramucosal gastric tumors using an insulated tip diathermic knife. Endoscopy 2001;33:221-6.

19. Pech O, May A, Rabenstein T, et al. Endoscopic resection of early esophageal cancer. Gut 2007;56:1625-34.

20. Andreas Adam, Joseph Ellul, Anthony F Watkinson, Bien Soo Tan, Robert A Morgan, Michael P Saunders, Robert C Mason. Palliation of inoperable Esophageal Carcinoma: a Prospective Randomized Trial of Laser Therapy and stent Placement. Radiology 1997;202:344-8.

21. Isaac Raijman. Expandable metal stents and other palliative techniques for esophageal malignancies. In Manoop S Bhutani, Rakesh K Tandon (Eds): Advances in Gastrointestinal Endoscopy 2001;6:86-102.

22. Guitron A, Adalid R, Huerta F, et al. Palliative treatment of esophageal cancer with endoscopic injection of alcohol. Rev Gastroenterol Mex 1996; 61:208-11.

23. Nwokolo CU, Payne-James JJ, Silk DB, et al. Palliation of malignant dysphagia by ethanol induced tumor necrosis. Gut 1994;35:299-303.
24. Freitas D, Gouveia H, Sofia C, et al. Endoscopic Nd:YAG laser therapy as palliative treatment for esophageal and cardial cancer. Hepatogastroenterology 1995;42:633-7.
25. Ahlquist DA, Gostout CJ, Viggiano TR, et al. Endoscopic laser palliation of malignant dysphagia: a prospective study. Mayo Clin Proc 1987;62:867-74.
26. De Palma GD, di Matteo E, Romano C, et al. Plastic prosthesis versus expandable metal stents for palliation of inoperable esophageal thoracic carcinoma: a controlled prospective study. Gastrointest Endosc 1996;43:478-82.
27. Mosca F, Consoli A, Stracqualvrsi A, et al. Our experience with the use of a plastic prosthesis and self-expanding stents in the palliative treatment of malignant neoplastic stenoses of the esophagus and cardia. Comparative analysis of results. Chin Ital 2002;54:341-50 Italian.
28. Knyrim K. Wagner HJ, Bethge N, et al. A controlled trial of an expansile metal stent for palliation of esophageal obstruction due to inoperable cancer. N Engl J Med 1993;329:1302-7.
29. Mosca F, Consoli A, Stracqualursi A, et al. Comparative retrospective study on the use of plastic prostheses and self-expanding metal stents in palliative treatment of malignant strictures of the esophagus and cardia. Dis Esophagus 2003;16:119-25.
30. Shimi SM. Self-expanding metallic stents in the management of advanced esophageal cancer: a review. Semin Laparosc Surg 2000;7:9-21.
31. Luis Carlos Sabbagh. Esophageal cancer. Gastrointest Endoscopy, 2009;69(2): 593-6.
32. Rene Lambert. Balancing the benefits and risks of esophageal stenting in the palliation of malignant dysphagia. The Journal of Supportive Oncology 2008;6(6):275-6.
33. Vakil N, Morris Al, Marcon N, et al. A prospective randomized controlled trial of covered expandable metal stents in the palliation of malignant esophageal obstruction at the gastroesophageal junction. Am J Gastroenterol 2001;96:1791-6.
34. Homs MY, Siersema PD. Stents in the GI tract. Expert Rev Med Devices 2007;4:741-52.
35. Els MI, Verschuur RN, Ernst J Kuipers, Peter D Siersema. Esophageal stents for malignant strictures close to the upper esophageal sphincter. Gastrointest Endoscopy 2007;66(6):1082-90.
36. Jin-He Guo, Gao-Jun Teng, Guang-Yu Zhu, Shi-Cheng He, Wen Fang, Gang Deng, Guo-Zhao Li. Self-expandable esophageal stent Loaded with [125]I Seeds: Initial Experience in patients with advanced Esophageal Cancer. Radiology 2008;247(2):574-81.
37. Churn M, Jones B, Myint AS, et al. Radical radiotherapy incorporating a brachytherapy boost for the treatment of cancer of thoracic esophagus: results from a cohort of patients and review of the literature. Clin Oncol (R Coll Radiol) 2002;14:117-22.
38. Homs MY, Steyerberg EW, Eijkenboom WM, et al. Single-dose brachytherapy versus metal stent placement for the palliation of dysphagia from esophageal cancer: multicenter randomized trial. Lancet 2004;364:1497-1504.

39. Allum WH, Griffin SM, Watson A, Colin Jones D. Guidelines for the management of esophageal and gastric cancer. Gut 2002;50(Suppl 5):V1-23.

40. Eriksen JR. Palliation of non-resectable carcinoma of cardia and esophagus by argon beam coagulation. Dan Med Bull 2002;49:346-9.

41. Heindroff H, Wojdemann M, Bisgaard T, Svendsen LB. Endoscopic palliation of inoperable cancer of the esophagus or cardia by argon electrocoagulation. Scand Gastroenterol 1998;33:21-3.

42. Jemal A, Tiwari RC, Murray T, et al. Cancer statistics 2004. CA Cancer. J Clin 2004;54:8-29.

43. Nix GA, Dubbelman C, Wilson JH, et al. Prognostic implications of tumor diameter in carcinoma of the head of the pancreas. Cancer 1991;67:529-35.

44. Todd H Baron. Palliation of malignant obstructive jaundice. Gastroenterol Clin N Am 2006;35:101-12.

45. Michael Saunders, Georgios I Papachristou, Kevin M McGrath, Adam Slivka. Endoscopic palliation of Pancreatic Cancer; Gastroenterol Clin N Am 2007; 36:455-76.

46. Soehendra N, Reynders-Frederix V. Palliative bile duct drainage: a new endoscopic method of introducing a transpapillary drain. Endoscopy 1980; 12:8-11.

47. Costamagna G, Pandolfi M. Endoscopic stenting for biliary and pancreatic malignancies. J Clin Gastroenterol 2004;38:59-67.

48. Groen AK, Out T, Huibregtse K, et al. Characterization of the content of occluded biliary endoprostheses. Endoscopy 1987;19:57-9.

49. Isayama H, Komatsu Y, Tsujino T, Sasahira N, Hirano K, Tada N, et al. A Prospective randomized study of "covered" versus "uncovered" diamond stents for management of distal malignant biliary obstruction. Gut 2004;53: 729-34.

50. Speer AG, Cotton PB, MacRac KD. Endoscopic management of malignant biliary obstruction. Stents of 10 French gauge are preferable to stents of 8 french gauge. Gastrointest Endosc 1988;34:412-7.

51. Pedersen FM. Endoscopic management of malignant biliary obstruction. Is stent size of 10 French gauge better than 7 french gauge? Scand J Gastroenterol 1993;28:185-9.

52. Pereira Lima J, Jakobs R, Maier M, et al. Endoscopic biliary stenting for the palliation of pancreatic cancer: results, survival predictive factors and comparison of 10 Fr with 11.5 Fr gauge stents. Am J Gastroenterol 1996; 91:2179-84.

53. Pietro Di Giorgio, Leonardo De Luca. Comparison of treatment outcomes between biliary plastic stent placement with and without endoscopic sphincterotomy for operable malignant common bile duct obstruction. World J Gastroenterol 2004;10(8):1212-4.

54. Tringali A, Mutignani M, Perri V, et al. A prospective randomized multi-center trial comparing Double layer and polyethylene stents for malignant distal common bile duct strictures. Endoscopy 2003;35:992-7.

55. Jason N Rogart, Ara Boghos, Federico Rossi, Hashem Al-Hashem, Uzma D Siddiqui, Priya Jamidar. Analysis of endoscopic management of occluded metal biliary stents at a single tertiary care center. Gastrointest Endoscopy 2008;68(4):676-82.

56. Mark S Choh, James A Madura II. The role of minimally invasive treatments in surgical oncology. Surg Clin N Am 2009;89:53-77.

57. Fukami N, Lee JH. Endoscopic treatment of large sessile and flat colorectal lesions. Curr Opin Gastroenterol 2006;22:54-9.

58. Kevin A Tolliver, Douglas K Rex. Colonoscopic Polypectomy; Gastroenterol Clin N Am 2008;37:229-51.

59. Levin TR, Zhao W, Conoll C, et al. Complications of colonoscopy in an integrated health care delivery system. Ann Intern Med 2006;145:880-6.

60. David M Poppers, Gregory B Haber. Endoscopic Mucosal Resection of Colonic lesions. Current Applications and Future Prospects. Med Clin Am 2008;92:687-705.

61. Srinivas R Puli, Yasuo Kakugawa, Takuji Gotoda, Daphne Antillon, Yutaka Saito, Mainor R Antillon. Meta-analysis and systematic review of colorectal endoscopic mucosal resection. World J Gastroenterol 2009;15(34):4273-7.

62. Fujishiro M, Yahagi N, Kakushima N, et al. Endoscopic submucosal dissection of esophageal squamous cell neoplasms. Clin Gastroenterol Hepatol 2006;4(6):688-94.

63. Horiuchi A, Maeyama H, Ochi Y, et al. Usefulness of Dennis colorectal tube in endoscopic decompression of acute, malignant colonic obstruction. Gastrointest Endosc 2001;54:229-32.

64. Jesùs Garcia-Cano, Ferran Gonzalez-Huix, Diego Juzgado, et al. Use of self-expanding metal stents to treat malignant obstruction in general endoscopic practice. Gastrointestinal Endoscopy 2006;64(6):914-20.

65. Carne PW, Fyre JN, Robertson GM, Frizelle FA. Stents or open operation for palliation of colorectal cancer: a retrospective, cohort study of perioperative outcome and long-term survival. Dis colon Rectum 2004;47:1455-61.

66. Johnson R, Marsh R, Corson J, Seymour K. A comparison of two methods of palliation of large bowel obstruction due to irremovable colon cancer. Ann R Coll Surg Engl 2004;86:99-103.

67. Lewin KJ, Appelman HD. Tumors of the esophagus and stomach. In Rosai J (Ed): Atlas of tumor pathology, 3rd series, fascicle 18. Armed Forces Institute of Pathology: Washington, DC, 1996.

68. Everett SM, Axon AT. Early Gastric cancer in Europe. Gut 1997;41:142-50.

69. Hisamichi S. Screening for gastric cancer. World J Surg 1989;13:31-7.

70. Sue-Ling HM, Martin I, Griffith J, et al. Early gastric cancer: 46 cases treated in one surgical department. Gut 33:1318-22.

71. Folli S, Dente M, Dell' A More, et al. Early gastric cancer: prognostic factors in 223 patients. Br J Surg 1995;82:952-6.

72. Makuchi H, Kise Y, Shimada H, et al. Endoscopic mucosal resection for early gastric cancer. Semin Surg Oncol 1999;17:108-16.

73. Ono H, Kondo H, Gotoda T, et al. Endoscopic mucosal resection for treatment of early gastric cancer. Gut 2001;48:225-9.

74. Hamada T, Kondo K, Itagaki Y, et al. Endoscopic mucosal resection for early gastric cancer. Nippon Rinsho 1996;54:1292-7.

75. Mizumoto S, Misumi A, Harada K, et al. Evaluation of endoscopic mucosal resection (EMR) as a curative therapy against early gastric cancer. Nippo Geka Gokkai Zasshi 1992;93:1071-4.

76. Gregory Y Lauwers, Shinichi Ban, Mari Mino, Shinichi ota, Takayuki Matsumo, Shin Arai, et al. Endoscopic mucosal resection for gastric epithelial neoplasms: a study of 39 cases with emphasis on evaluation of specimens and recommendations for optimal pathologic analysis. Modern Pathology 2004;17:2-8.

77. Chun-Chao-Chang, I-Lin Lee, Peng–Jen Chen, Hsui-Powang, et al. Endoscopic submucosal dissection for gastric epithelial tumors: a multicenter study in Taiwan. J Formos Med Assoc 2009;108(1):38-44.

78. Mark Topazian, Todd H Baron. Endoscopic fenestration of duodenal stents using argon plasma to facilitate ERCP; Gastrointestinal Endoscopy 2009;9(1):166-9.

SECTION SIX

VASCULAR

CHAPTER TWELVE

Endovascular Repair of
Abdominal Aortic Aneurysms

Isuru S Nammuni, Jonathan R Boyle

INTRODUCTION

Over the last 40 years, the prevalence of abdominal aortic aneurysms (AAA) has steadily increased. The vast majority of AAAs are asymptomatic until they rupture. Despite major medical advances during this period, the overall mortality after rupture remains as high as 80%. The aim is, therefore, to detect and repair these aneurysms electively to evade this high mortality.

Since the advent of endovascular aneurysm repair (EVAR) by Parodi et al in 1991,[1] EVAR has revolutionized elective aneurysm repair, with significant decreases in operative mortality. EVAR is also increasingly being used for repair of ruptured abdominal aortic aneurysms (RAAAs) with encouraging results. It is clear that EVAR is a continually evolving field, which is vastly changing the practice of vascular surgery.

SCREENING

Since the majority of AAAs are asymptomatic, most aneurysms are incidentally found on clinical examination or on imaging performed for other abdominal pathology. Various efforts have been made to investigate the benefits of a screening program in increasing detection of AAA in the population. Three large scale population-based randomized controlled trials[2-4] have shown a clear decrease in mortality for screened males > 65 years old. In response to this, several national screening programs have been introduced. The UK National Screening Program aims to invite all men to be screened with ultrasound at the age of 65. If an AAA is detected, these men are followed with ultrasound and the AAA is repaired once it reaches an appropriate size. This will most certainly increase the number of aneurysms repaired electively and hence, have a positive impact on future mortality rates due to ruptured AAA.

Key Point

- Population screening with ultrasound for men > 65 is cost-effective and improves survival.

INDICATIONS FOR EVAR

Since elective AAA repair is essentially a prophylactic operation, the decision to treat is a balance between the risks associated with rupture and operative risks. Two multicenter trials (ADAM, UK Small Aneurysm Trial)[5,6] showed there was no survival benefit in open repair for aneurysms smaller than 5.5 cm diameter. It has been suggested, however, that the threshold for endovascular treatment may be different, given EVAR has a much lower operative mortality (1 to 2%) as compared to open repair (4 to 5%).[7,8] We currently await the results of two randomized controlled trials investigating the merit of EVAR in small aneurysms,[9,10] but in the interim most use the accepted threshold for intervention of 5.5 cm in men and 5 cm in women.

Key Point

- EVAR has the same size threshold for intervention as open repair (5.5 cm for men and 5.0 cm for women).

INFRARENAL ENDOVASCULAR ANEURYSM REPAIR

In 1991, Parodi et al[1] reported the first successful endovascular exclusion of an abdominal aortic aneurysm by implanting a dacron tube mounted on balloon-expandable stents. Since then, many commercially available stent grafts have been developed. Numerous problems with early stent grafts (stent fracture, fabric porosity and tears and stent migration) have led to the development of second and third generation stent grafts. Current generation stent grafts are bifurcated with varying methods of proximal fixation (infrarenal vs suprarenal with or without anchoring barbs) and modular design to allow for maximum versatility. They are made of either dacron or expanded polytetrafluoroethylene (ePTFE) fabric, supported by stainless steel or nitinol self-expanding stents. Various design improvements in stent grafts, delivery systems and techniques have led to a vast increase in the number of aneurysms amenable to endovascular management. The anatomical requirements for the currently available devices are summarized in Table 12.1.

Proximal Neck

A suitable proximal neck is crucial in achieving adequate seal and fixation of the endograft. The infrarenal neck is the portion of aorta between the lowest renal artery and the beginning of the aneurysmal segment. Due to advances in stent design, it is now possible to treat necks as short as 10 mm and angulation up to 75 degrees before reaching the limits of the manufacturers' indications for use.

TABLE 12.1

Anatomical requirements for endovascular aneurysm repair (EVAR)

Proximal neck	
• Neck length	> 10-15 mm
• Neck diameter	18-32 mm
• Suprarenal angulation	< 60°
• Infrarenal angulation	< 70°
• Presence of thrombus	No excessive thrombus to prevent fixation
• Flaring	Flaring < 10% of diameter over 15 mm length
Distal neck diameter	> 18-20 mm
Common iliac vessel	
• CIA length	> 10-15 mm
• CIA diameter	8-25 mm
Access vessels	
• EIA diameter	> 5.5-7 mm

Adaptation from Medtronic Endurant, Cook Zenith Flex and Gore Excluder indications for use.[35-37]

Access Vessels

Endovascular grafts are introduced through the iliac vessels and into the abdominal aorta via femoral artery cut down or percutaneous puncture. Focal iliac stenoses can be angioplastied to accommodate the graft delivery system, but if the overall caliber is inadequate this will preclude EVAR. If there is excessive iliac tortuosity and calcification, then this will also prevent the graft from being introduced into the aorta. Although new low profile, flexible, hydrophilic-coated delivery systems have been developed to combat this, occasionally an iliac conduit is required to enable the most tortuous vessels to be navigated. Some have alternatively placed long covered stents into small stenotic iliacs as "in situ" iliac conduits. These are then post-dilated to a size adequate to introduce the endovascular device.

Suprarenal Aneurysms

Branched and fenestrated aortic grafts have been developed to combat suprarenal and juxtarenal aneurysms with inadequate infrarenal necks. These are custom-made grafts manufactured according to the exact anatomical site of each aortic visceral branch. This fenestrated segment is then combined with smaller covered stents, which are used to bridge from the main stent into the branch vessels (Fig. 12.1). These endograft procedures are technically demanding and are usually reserved for patients who are not suitable for an open repair due to a hostile abdomen

173

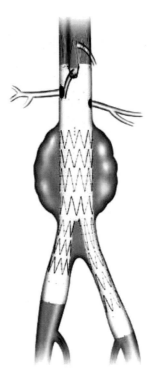

Fig. 12.1: Cook fenestrated aortic device.[35]

or recurrent aneurysms. Alternatively, a hybrid approach may be used in which visceral vessels are re-vascularized by grafts arising from the external iliac artery in a stage one laparotomy. As a second stage procedure, an endovascular stent is then placed from the supraceliac aorta, across the original visceral vessel origins and down into both common iliac vessels. This hybrid approach has also been employed to treat thoraco-abdominal aneurysms and dissections and combined with various arch vessel bypasses and de-branching procedures.

Iliac Branch Devices

Every attempt should be made to preserve the internal iliac arteries when performing endovascular stenting to prevent buttock claudication, erectile dysfunction and the risk of ischemia to pelvic organs.[11] However, if the common iliac vessels are too short or there is iliac aneurysmal disease present, this may not be possible with conventional stenting. Iliac branched devices have, therefore, been developed (Fig. 12.2). This involves stenting from the common iliac to the external iliac with a branch extending into the internal iliac artery. An additional covered stent is then used in a similar way to branched aortic devices to span into the internal iliac vessel and achieve a seal. This is then combined with a conventional bifurcated aortic stent to complete the aneurysm repair.

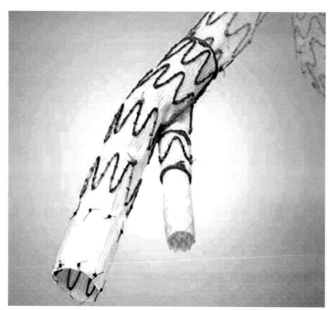

Fig. 12.2: Cook iliac branched device.[35]

Key Points

- Key anatomical considerations for EVAR are infrarenal neck length, angulation, and iliac aneurysm, occlusive disease or tortuosity.
- Every effort should be made to preserve the internal iliac arteries.

STENT COMPLICATIONS

Various concerns have been raised about the long-term durability of endovascular repair. Unlike an open repair, where the aneurysm is completely excluded from the circulation and the graft is sutured in place, the endovascular stent relies on the maintenance of position and aneurysm morphology to prevent sac re-pressurization and rupture. Complications, such as stent migration, kinking and endoleaks have been said to occur in 10 to 30% of patients[12-15] and predispose to late aneurysm rupture.

Stent Migration

Stent migration occurs when, over time, the stent moves from its original deployment location. Migration at the proximal end can occur, if the stent slips down the neck and into the aneurysm sac. This was a problem associated with the earlier endografts and the newest generation grafts incorporate suprarenal bare metal struts and fixation hooks or barbs to attempt to prevent this, although we are yet to see long-term results of these new grafts. Migration of the distal end of the endograft, with limbs retracting out of the common iliac arteries and into the sac and migration with disconnection of modular segments of the graft can also occur. **175**

Stent Fracture and Kinking

Fracture of the metal stents has also been a problem in the past. Newer, more conformable stent material, such as nitinol, and improved stent designs have become available although loss of column strength of the endograft and subsequent kinking and occlusion of limbs is still a concern.

Endoleak

An endoleak develops when there is perfusion of the aneurysm sac outside the stent graft.[16] Table 12.2 shows the various types of endoleak.[17] It was initially thought that all endoleaks were significant. We now recognize, however, that this is not necessarily the case. Type I and III endoleaks result in re-pressurization of the anuerysmal sac and therefore, need secondary interventions. This is often in the form of ancillary endovascular procedures, such as insertion of a proximal endograft cuff or Palmaz bare metal stent or a bridging stent graft to span the gap between disconnected or retracted limbs. Type II endoleaks, however, are a low-pressure leak and therefore, can usually be managed expectantly. If there is any increase in sac size on serial follow-up, this is an indication to intervene, as a change in the aneurysm morphology may lead to the development of one of the above complications and eventual rupture. A variety of methods have been devised to address Type II endoleaks, including transarterial or translumbar embolization of lumbar arteries with coils or ethylene vinyl alcohol copolymer (Onyx) and laparoscopic or extra-peritoneal ligation of feeding vessels with varying results.[18] Type IV endoleaks require re-lining of the endograft, and the concept of "Endotension" where the sac size increases without a demonstrable endoleak, remains a management quandary.

TABLE 12.2

Classification of endoleak[17]

Endoleak		
Type I	Attachment site leak	
• Type Ia	• Proximal attachment	
• Type Ib	• Distal attachment	
• Type Ic	• Iliac plug site	
Type II	Branch vessels (e.g. lumbar or IMA)	
• Type IIa	• Single vessel	
• Type IIb	• Multiple inflow and outflow vessels	
Type III	Graft defect	
• Type IIIa	• Modular junction leaks/disconnection	
• Type IIIb	• Graft fabric tear	
Type IV	Graft fabric porosity	
Endotension	Increase in sac size with no demonstrable leak	

With time, as stent graft technology improves and our medium- and long-term experience with EVAR grows, we expect the complication and secondary intervention rates to decline.

Key Points

- Fabric failure and stent fractures are uncommon with modern devices.
- All type I and type III endoleaks require intervention.
- Most type II endoleaks can be managed expectantly.

EVAR FOLLOW-UP

It is clear from the potential complications after EVAR that close surveillance needs to be maintained in order to detect complications and reduce the risk of late aneurysm ruptures. This is in contrast to open aneurysm repair after which patients are very rarely subjected to close long-term follow-up. There is little argument that contrast CT is the imaging modality of choice in preoperative planning for EVAR. However, for postoperative surveillance, the decision is not so clear cut. Since EVAR patients require repeated, ongoing investigations, issues of cumulative radiation dose and repeated contrast related renal injury[19] need to be considered, not to mention cost. A number of alternatives to contrast CT have, therefore, been suggested.

Duplex Ultrasound

The use of Duplex Ultrasound in screening and surveillance of asymptomatic AAA has been widely accepted. It has been shown to have a comparable sensitivity and specificity to CT in determining aneurysm sac size. It is not as sensitive in detecting specific endoleaks after EVAR, however, it is only the endoleaks associated with an increase in sac size that need intervention and therefore, duplex can be just as effective as contrast CT in determining which patients will ultimately require secondary intervention. In addition, contrast-enhanced ultrasound scanning (CEUS) is emerging as a method of detecting specific endoleaks. This technique employs intravenous injection of a microbubble contrast medium, which enhances visualization of blood flow and endoleaks. Second generation contrast media, which employ harmonic resonance further enhance image quality and evidence is emerging that this may even be more sensitive than CT at detecting low-flow endoleaks,[20] however, this is not yet widely available. Since it is often difficult to appreciate stent location and anatomy on serial ultrasound scans, duplex imaging is combined with plain radiographs to check for graft migration and limb kinking or disconnection.

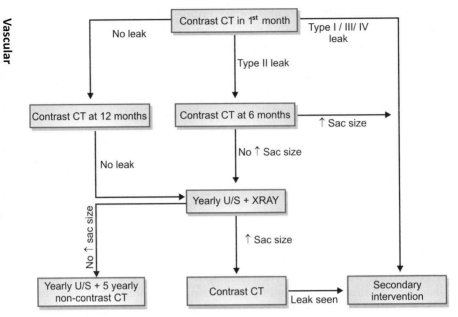

Fig. 12.3: Algorithm for postoperative surveillance following endovascular aneurysm repair.

Imaging Interval

In recent years, there has been a lot of debate as to the best regimen for performing these follow-up investigations. As we are only just starting to see medium- and long-term results of the few randomized controlled trials, it is difficult to know what is the best modality at each interval. The American Society of Vascular Surgeons recommendations published in their 2009 Guidelines[21] are summarized in Figure 12.3.

Key Point

- If no concerning endoleaks and increase in sac size are found in the first year, ongoing surveillance with ultrasound and plain radiographs is adequate.

LONG-TERM RESULTS

Aside from numerous case series and cohort studies, we currently have two large multicenter, randomized controlled trials and two large population databases, which are reporting medium- to long-term data. We know that EVAR is associated with a significant reduction in 30-day mortality as compared to open repair (1.6% vs 4%).[12-15] This survival benefit, however, was not shown to persist past 1 year and the all-cause mortality was no different to open repair after 4 years (28%).[14]

The five-year results of the dutch randomized endovascular aneurysm management (DREAM) Trial have now been presented[22] and suggest the outcomes may even be worse for the EVAR group in the long term. This is quite a disconcerting finding as it challenges our previous views regarding the benefits of EVAR. Various reasons have been put forward to explain this.

Aneurysm-related Mortality

Aneurysm related deaths during follow-up remain low in the EVAR group (around 1% per year) and are mainly related to stent migration and endoleak.[19] It is clear that ensuring patients are compliant with ongoing surveillance programs after EVAR is of paramount importance, if we are to reduce this late aneurysm-related death rate.

Cardiovascular Mortality

Deaths from cardiovascular disease are the leading cause of non-aneurysm-related mortality after aneurysm repair. It was previously thought that the physiologically more demanding open repair simply unmasked underlying cardiovascular disease, leading to a higher operative mortality. The EVAR patients manifested the same underlying cardiovascular disease a few years later, as a "catch-up effect." In light of the new data, which suggest that mortality five years after EVAR exceeds that of open repair, alternative explanations have been put forward.

Following EVAR, the aneurysm sac thromboses and potentially remains in contact with the circulation, especially in the presence of an ongoing endoleak. A recent study has shown that there are elevated levels of cytokines such as interleukin-6, which has been identified as a risk factor for cardiovascular and all-cause mortality.[23]

Renal Dysfunction

Evidence suggests that there is a decline in renal function in the long-term following EVAR.[19] The etiology of this effect is likely to be multi-factorial. EVAR patients receive repeated nephrotoxic contrast administration during follow-up CT scanning and secondary interventions to treat endoleaks. Various strategies have been used to protect from contrast nephropathy in patients with established renal impairment, however, there is a lack of evidence to support these. In addition, these measures are currently not applied to patients with normal renal function and it has been suggested that we should give renal protection to all patients undergoing postoperative EVAR surveillance with iodine contrast. A shift away from contrast CT and the increasing importance of non-nephrotoxic contrast-enhanced ultrasound will also certainly have a positive impact.

Suprarenal fixation of the device is another potential cause of long-term decline in renal function. Suprarenal fixation involves the projection of bare metal struts across the renal ostia, predisposing to renal artery emboli and complete occlusion. Several small studies have suggested that suprarenal fixation is harmless, however, a recent meta-analysis of the available data indicated that this may not be the case.[24]

Key Points

- EVAR has significantly lower procedural mortality than open aneurysm repair.
- EVAR has equivalent mortality to open repair in the medium term.
- Long-term results are unknown with current devices and endovascular practices.

EVAR FOR RUPTURED ANEURYSMS

Over the last 40 years, despite advances in emergency surgical services and postoperative care, there has only been a modest improvement in outcomes for ruptured abdominal aortic aneurysms. The mortality rates for patients surviving to hospital are still in the order of 50%. Although the introduction of EVAR in 1991 has revolutionized elective aneurysm surgery, we have not seen a similar adoption rate for the emergency setting. This is surprising, given that the benefits of a physiologically less demanding approach would seem to be the greatest for rupture patients. Centers which have adopted an aggressive emergency EVAR (eEVAR) protocol have achieved exceptional results with mortality rates as low as 13%.[25] Perhaps the slow adoption rate is due to various logistic reasons, since providing an endovascular service for ruptured aneurysms requires a large assortment of graft sizes available on site, not to mention the availability of endovascular interventionists and ancillary staff. Aside from these practicalities, various factors need consideration when treating ruptured aneurysms with EVAR.

Patient Selection

Numerous scoring systems, such as the Hardman Index, V-POSSUM and Glasgow Aneurysm Score, have been devised to predict the outcome for individual rupture patients undergoing open repair. A recent meta-analysis, however, has highlighted that these scoring systems cannot simply be applied to emergency EVAR (eEVAR), as patients with similar comorbidities have a lower mortality rate following EVAR as compared to open repair.[26] It is therefore suggested that until more conclusive evidence is available, those patients who would not undergo open repair on account of co-morbidities, should be offered EVAR.

Preoperative Management

The improvements in survival in recently reported series have been partly attributed to the concept of hypotensive hemostasis. This is based on the premise that a low blood pressure maintains integrity of the hematoma formed around the rupture site and temporarily prevents further blood loss. Blood pressures as low as 50-70 mm Hg are tolerated, provided there is no evidence of cerebral hypoperfusion. Restriction of intravenous fluids is essential, and some centers even suggest active lowering of BP below 90 mm Hg.[25]

Aortic balloon occlusion may be required to achieve hemodynamic stability in the case of free rupture. A compliant aortic balloon is inserted into the supraceliac aorta via either a femoral or a brachial cut-down and inflated to occlude the aorta and achieve hemostatic control. This maneuver can often be performed in a matter of minutes, provided the radiological facilities are on hand. This means that even the most unstable patients who have in the past been rushed straight to theater, can be rapidly stabilized and assessed for EVAR.

Imaging

Contrast CT is undoubtedly the gold standard for preoperative planning and device selection for eEVAR. Since the vast majority of patients with a ruptured aneurysm survive the first two hours following presentation to hospital, most patients can be safely imaged.[27] In addition, the concept of hypotensive hemostasis has meant that patients who were traditionally thought of as "too unstable to go to the scanner" are now considered optimally managed. Some have also suggested that adequate imaging for EVAR planning can be obtained with on-table angiography in the most unstable of patients.[28]

Anesthetic

The minimally invasive endovascular approach should be carried out under local anesthesia where possible. This avoids the hemodynamic changes associated with general or spinal anesthesia and may reduce postoperative respiratory complications. Local anesthetic is used to facilitate bilateral groin cut-down; however, this requires a cooperative patient who is able to lie still and stop breathing at the relevant stages to allow adequate imaging and stent positioning. In the case of aorto-uni-iliac (AUI) devices, the aneurysm is initially excluded under local anesthesia and the patient can subsequently be anesthetized to allow tunneling and clamping for a femoro-femoral crossover, if this is not tolerated under local anesthesia.

Anatomical Considerations

The basic anatomical requirements for elective EVAR apply for the emergency setting with a few adaptations. Unlike in the elective setting where grafts can be obtained specific to the patient's requirements, acute ruptures require repair with what is available on hand. AUI devices provide the greatest amount of flexibility, as they can be adapted to almost any length of aneurysm. A few differing proximal neck diameters, combined with a selection of limb extensions and a few standard iliac occlusion plugs will be able to treat the majority of aneurysms. In addition, an AUI achieves exclusion of the aneurysm most expediently, as there is no need for cannulation of the contralateral limb. A femoro-femoral crossover is required in these instances, although this can be performed in a more controlled fashion, as once the AUI has been deployed, there is no risk of hemodynamic instability.

It is also noted that the strict anatomical requirements for EVAR are often not closely adhered to in the case of ruptured aneurysms. Often patients who would not be offered an EVAR electively due to non-ideal anatomy are offered EVAR for a rupture if the risks of open repair are too great. This may account for the higher rate of graft complications seen with EVAR for ruptures, with some reports of a 25% endoleak rate and 15% re-intervention rate.[29]

Outcomes

There is a lack of good quality level 1 evidence regarding the efficacy of EVAR for ruptured AAA, however, the initial results seem very encouraging. A recent meta-analysis of all available non-randomized data on EVAR for ruptured AAA[30] showed a pooled mortality of only 29% while another meta-analysis showed a significant reduction in intra-operative blood loss, intensive care stay and overall hospital stay.[31] There are currently three multicenter randomized controlled trials in progress, (AJAX, IMPROVE, ECAR trials)[32-34] which aim to provide more conclusive evidence as to the merits of providing an endovascular treatment option for ruptured aneurysms.

Key Points

- EVAR for ruptured aneurysms appears to improve outcomes.
- No scoring systems have been validated for patients undergoing emergency EVAR.
- Hypotensive hemostasis is an important part of preoperative management.
- Often a compromise must be made between anatomical requirements and the graft sizes available on hand.
- Local anesthesia should be used whenever possible.

CONCLUSION

It is clear that endovascular aneurysm repair is a rapidly advancing area of vascular surgery. As endografts continue to be improved and our long-term experience grows, EVAR is sure to have a positive impact on mortality rates for aneurysmal disease.

REFERENCES

1. Parodi JC, Palmaz JC, Baron HD, et al. Transfemoral intraluminal graft implantation for abdominal aortic aneurysm. Ann Vasc Surg 1991;5:491-9.
2. Ashton HA, Buxton MJ, Day NE, et al. The Multicentre Aneurysm Screening Study (MASS) into the effect of abdominal aortic aneurysm screening on mortality in men: a randomised controlled trial. Lancet 2002;360:1531-9.
3. Lindholt J, Juul S, Fasting H, et al. Screening for abdominal aortic aneurysms: single-centre randomised controlled trial. Br Med J 2005;330:750-4.
4. Norman PE, Jamrozik K, Lawrence Brown MM, et al. Population-based randomised controlled trial on impact of screening on mortality from abdominal aortic aneurysm. Br Med J 2004;329:1259-62.
5. Lederle FA, Wilson SE, Johnson GR, et al. Immediate repair compared with surveillance of small abdominal aortic aneurysms. N Eng J Med 2002;346: 1437-44.
6. The United Kingdom Small Aneurysm Trial Participants. Long-term outcomes of immediate repair compared with surveillance of small abdominal aortic aneurysms. N Eng J Med 2002;346:1445-52.
7. The EVAR Trial Participants. Comparison of endovascular aneurysm repair with open repair in patients with abdominal aortic aneurysm (EVAR trial 1) 30-day operative mortality: randomised controlled trial. Lancet 2004; 364:843-8.
8. Prinssen M, Verhoeven EL, Buth J, et al. A randomised trial comparing conventional and endovascular repair of abdominal aortic aneurysm. N Eng J Med 2004;351:1607-18.
9. Cao P. CAESAR trial collaborators. Comparison of surveillance vs aortic endografting for small aneurysm repair (CAESAR) trial: study design and progress. Eur J Vasc Endovasc Surg 2005;30:245-51.
10. Ouriel K. The PIVOTAL study: A randomised comparison of endovascular repair versus surveillance in patients with smaller abdominal aortic aneurysms. J Vasc Surg 2009;49:266-9.
11. Rayt HS, Brown MJ, Lambert KV, et al. Buttock Claudication and Erectile Dysfunction After Internal Iliac Artery Embolisation in Patients Prior to Endovascular Aortic Aneurysm Repair. Cardiovasc Intervent Radiol 2008; 31:728-34.
12. Thomas SM, Gaines PA, Barone JD, et al. Results from the prospective registry of endovascular treatment of abdominal aortic aneurysms (RETA): Mid-term results to five years. Eur J Vasc Endovasc Surg 2005;29:563-70.
13. Blankensteijn JD, De Jong S, Prinssen M, et al. Two year outcomes after conventional or endovascular repair of abdominal aortic aneurysms. N Engl J Med 2005;352:2398-2405.
14. The EVAR Trial Participants. Endovascular aneurysm repair versus open repair in patients with abdominal aortic aneurysm (EVAR trial 1): randomised controlled trial. Lancet 2005;365:2179-86.

15. Buth J, Hobo R and EUROSTAR collaborators. Secondary interventions following endovascular abdominal aortic aneurysm repair using current endografts. A EUROSTAR report. J Vasc Surg 2006;43:896-902.

16. White GH, Yu W, May J, et al. Endoleak as a complication of endoluminal grafting of abdominal aortic aneurysms: Classification, incidence, diagnosis and management. J Endovasc Surg 1997;4:152-68.

17. Veith FJ, Baum RA, Ohki T, et al. Nature and significance of endoleaks and endotension: Summary of opinions expressed at an international conference. J Vasc Surg 2002;35:1029-35.

18. Green MG, Rose RJ. Endoleak management following Endovascular Aneurysm Repair. J Vasc Interv Radiol 2008;19:S37-S43.

19. Walsh SR, Tang TY, Boyle JR. Renal consequences of endovascular abdominal aortic aneurysm repair. J Vasc Endovasc Ther 2008;15:73-82.

20. Napoli V, Bargellini I, Sardella SG, et al. Abdominal aortic aneurysm: contrast-enhanced US for missed endoleaks after endoluminal repair. Radiology 2004;233:217-25.

21. Chaikof EL, Brewster DC, Dalman RL, et al. SVS practice guidelines for the care of patients with an abdominal aortic aneurysm: Executive summary. J Vasc Surg 2009;50:880-96.

22. Blankensteijn JD. Shocking and unexpected 5-year results from the DREAM trial. Veith Symposium 2008;XIV.08.

23. Choke E, Cockerill GW, Loftus IM, Thompson MM, Dawson JA. The long-term effects of open and endovascular aneurysm repair on circulating interleukin-6. Eur J Vasc Endovasc Surg 2009;37:43-5.

24. Walsh SR, Boyle JR, Lynch AG, et al. Suprarenal endograft fixation and medium-term renal function: systematic review and meta-analysis. J Vasc Surg 2008;47:1364-70.

25. Mayer D, Pfammatter T, Rancic Z, et al. 10 years of emergency endovascular aneurysm repair for ruptured abdominal aortoiliac aneurysms: Lessons learned. Ann Surg 2009;249:510-5.

26. Karkos CD, Karamanos D, Papazoglou KO, et al. Usefulness of the Hardman Index in predicting outcome after endovascular repair of ruptured abdominal aortic aneurysms. J Vasc Surg 2008;48:788-94.

27. Lloyd GM, Brown MJ, Norwood MGA, et al. Feasibility of preoperative computer tomography in patients with ruptured abdominal aortic aneurysm: A time to death study in patients without operation. J Vasc Surg 2004;39: 788-91.

28. Ohki T, Veith FJ. Endovascular grafts and other image-guided catheter based adjuncts to improve the treatment of ruptured aortoiliac aneurysms. Ann Surg 2000;4:466-79.

29. Oranen BI, Bos WTGJ, Verhoeven ELG, et al. Is emergency endovascular aneurysm repair associated with higher secondary intervention risk at mid-term follow-up? J Vasc Surg 2006;44:1156-61.

30. Harkin DW, Giannakou A, Gerassimidis TS, Karkos CD. Mortality after endovascular repair of ruptured abdominal aortic aneurysms. A systematic review and meta-analysis. Arch Surg 2009;144:770-8.

31. Sadat U, Boyle JR, Walsh SR, et al. Endovascular vs open repair of acute abdominal aortic aneurysms. A systematic review and meta-analysis. J Vasc Surg 2008;48:227-36.

32. Amsterdam Acute Aneurysm Trial Collaborators. Amsterdam Acute Aneurysm Trial: Background Design and Methods. Vascular 2006;14:1-6.
33. Powell JT. Time to IMPROVE the management of ruptured abdominal aortic aneurysm: IMPROVE Trialists. Eur J Vasc Endovasc Surg 2009;38:237-8.
34. ECAR trial. www.clinicaltrials.gov NCT00577616
35. COOK Medical, Boomington IN. Zenith Flex AAA Endovascular Graft instructions for use. www.cookmedical.com
36. MEDTRONIC, Minneapolis MN. The Endurant Stent Graft System Instructions for Use. www.medtronic.com
37. GORE Medical, Flagstaff AZ. Gore Excluder AAA Endoprosthesis Instructions for Use. www.goremedical.com

CHAPTER■ THIRTEEN

Management of
Vascular Injuries

Andrew L Tambyraja, Roderick TA Chalmers

INTRODUCTION

The epidemiology of vascular trauma has changed in recent years. An increase in civilian violence and high-energy accidents has been coupled with an increase in major vascular trauma.[1] Penetrating vascular trauma may result in vessel laceration or transection, vascular thrombosis, active hemorrhage, traumatic arterio-venous fistulation or pseudoaneurysm formation. Blunt trauma may cause disruption of the tunica intima, resulting in tears or dissection or even complete transmural rupture. Aortic and central vascular injury is a life-threatening event, often associated with multisystem injury and death. Peripheral vascular injury is less life threatening but is associated with a considerable degree of limb loss and disability. Military vascular injuries are largely due to high velocity missiles and blast injuries. By contrast, civilian injuries are most commonly due to penetrating knife wounds or low-velocity handgun shots and blunt injury from road traffic accidents. Despite these discrepancies, recent advances in the understanding and management of vascular trauma continue to stem largely from experience on the battlefield.

RESUSCITATION

The morbid effects of vascular injuries are mediated by hemorrhage and/ or direct end-organ ischemia. The physiological homeostatic mechanisms that aim to counter these effects are underpinned by the interplay of vasospasm, hypotension and hemostasis. Arterial injury is accompanied by local vasospasm that coupled with low blood pressure, promotes the formation of a stable clot to arrest blood loss. This premise is central to the concept of damage control resuscitation– permissive hypotension and the prevention of hypothermia and coagulopathy.

The evidence to support hypotensive resuscitation stems from urban trauma series and has been reinforced by contemporary military data.[2,3] Such a strategy is reported to improve the survival of hypotensive patients with penetrating truncal injury. Resuscitation to a systolic blood pressure of 70 mm Hg versus 100 mm Hg resulted in no difference in mortality in patients with blunt or penetrating injuries.[3] In a military context, fluid resuscitation is restrictively titrated to achieve a radial pulse and adequate cerebral perfusion.[4] American military series have recommended high molecular weight colloid solutions as the preferred intravenous fluid for resuscitation. Resuscitation with such solutions has been shown to result in a reduction in the volume requirement when compared to crystalloid solution in animal models of hemorrhagic shock.[5] They are also shown to reduce blood loss and improve coagulation profiles in hypovolemic patients undergoing major surgery.[6]

In severely injured patients, coagulopathy induced by trauma may occur due to the loss and dilution of components of the clotting cascade, hypothermia and acidosis. However, the novel concept of acute traumatic coagulopathy is now recognized in up to 25% of patients.[7] Acute traumatic coagulopathy is directly induced by trauma and shock and propagated by tissue hypoperfusion, causing systemic activation of the anticoagulant protein C pathway. The concept of hemostatic resuscitation mandates a proactive policy of simultaneously restoring tissue perfusion and correcting coagulopathy. Traditional transfusion practices are challenged and coagulation products should be given early with a close ratio to transfused red blood cells. Evidence to support this practice exists from military and civilian series and existing military protocols advocate a 1:1:1 ratio of fresh frozen plasma, platelets and red blood cells.[8-10] However, safe transfusion practice is governed by minimizing patient exposure to allogeneic blood products wherever possible. Immediate point of care functional testing of coagulation, such as thromboelastometry and thomboelastography, can greatly inform transfusion strategies and minimize unnecessary transfusion while guiding specific blood product replacement more precisely.

Recombinant factor VIIa (rFVIIa) has been shown to reduce blood loss in animal models of hemorrhage.[11] In prospective randomized trials, it also has been shown to reduce blood loss and transfusions after elective surgery.[12] In a prospective randomized trial performed in trauma patients, rFVIIa use resulted in a reduction in red blood cell transfusion after blunt trauma with a similar trend seen in penetrating trauma.[13] These results have been reinforced by military data, which showed that early rFVIIa use could reduce red blood cell transfusion in a cohort of patients with primarily penetrating injuries.[14]

Key Points

- The lethal triad of hypothermia, acidosis and coagulopathy should be avoided in patients with vascular injuries.
- Coagulopathy should be treated aggressively with blood products and supported by near patient testing wherever possible.
- Permissive hypotension can reduce blood loss and improve coagulation profiles.

ASSESSMENT

When accompanied by an appropriate mechanism of injury, the cardinal clinical signs of vascular injury are active hemorrhage, expanding hematoma, distal ischemia, the presence of an underlying bruit or thrill or neurological deficit. In addition, an ankle brachial pressure index of < 0.9 can be used to augment clinical assessment for arterial injury.

One or more of these positive findings is an indication for further investigation or direct intervention. The traditional approach to the management of vascular injuries has been one of direct surgical exploration in the unstable patient with strong signs of vascular injury or preliminary diagnostic radiological investigation. With the increased scope of endovascular intervention, it has become desirable to obtain arterial imaging whenever feasible. Traditional teaching recommends the use of contrast angiography as the gold standard investigation. The merits of this approach are significant, in that it can facilitate synchronous endovascular therapy. However, this must be weighed against the invasive nature of the examination and the possibility of a negative investigation, the considerable time taken to acquire necessary diagnostic detail and the poor cost-effectiveness profile.[15,16] Recently, there has been a move towards noninvasive imaging modalities, such as computed tomography (CT), duplex and magnetic resonance imaging (MRI). Of these, multi-row detector computed tomography (MDCT) has established itself as the first line investigation of choice when dealing with isolated vascular injuries or the multiply injured patient. MDCT permits rapid primary radiological survey with targeted imaging as required. With the newer generation of 64-MDCT, such an investigation can be performed in a matter of seconds with relatively modest doses of intravenous contrast and ionizing radiation compared to earlier scanners. Information on the location, extent and nature of injuries is quickly acquired and allows vascular injuries to be triaged into the management options of observation, endovascular intervention and open surgical intervention (Fig. 13.1). The validity of CT angiography, when compared with contrast angiography, is reported to have a sensitivity and specificity in detecting arterial injuries of between 90 and 100%.[16,17] Discordant clinical findings and CT angiography or trying to distinguish acute arterial vasospasm from subtle arterial injuries, can be further clarified by direct angiography as and when necessary.

Key Point

- MDCT is increasingly used as a first line radiological investigation in the assessment of trauma.

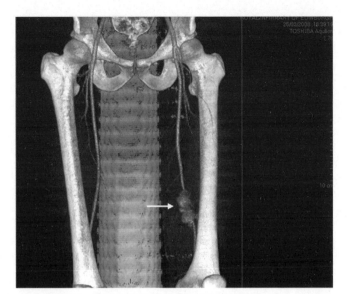

Fig. 13.1: CT angiogram of left superficial artery false aneurysm caused by penetrating injury.

ENDOVASCULAR STRATEGIES

The major recent paradigm shift in the management of vascular injuries has been the application of endovascular interventions. The ability to control and treat vascular injuries without direct open surgical exposure of distorted traumatized tissues, in anatomical locations potentially difficult to access, is highly desirable. Furthermore, the lesser magnitude of physiological insult associated with an endovascular approach, compared to an open procedure is attractive in the multiply injured patient. In its simplest form, endovascular intervention may take the form of the use of balloon occlusion catheters to achieve immediate, but temporary control of active hemorrhage. Catheters passed from the femoral artery can be used to deploy an occlusion balloon proximal to the source of bleeding. This can allow a period of restorative resuscitation before definitive surgical or endovascular therapy is undertaken. An inflated balloon can also serve as a useful landmark in guiding surgical exploration.

Key Point

- Endovascular techniques provide a useful therapeutic modality in the temporary and definitive management of some vascular injuries.

Aortic Injuries

In the United Kingdom, aortic trauma accounts for about 0.3% of cases admitted to hospital; this figure is up to 10 times greater in the USA.[18]

Vascular

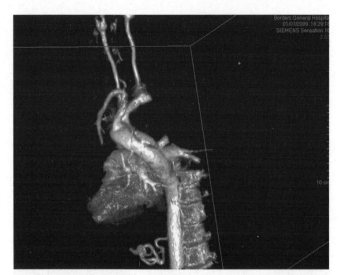

Fig. 13.2: CT angiogram of blunt traumatic dissection of proximal descending thoracic aorta.

Blunt injury secondary to deceleration is the most common mecahanism of injury to the thoracic aorta and great vessels. Traumatic shearing forces are greatest at points of aortic fixation: the atrial attachment of the pulmonary veins and vena cava, the ligamentum arteriosum and the diaphragm. The most common site for aortic injury is the proximal descending aorta beyond the left subclavian artery (Fig. 13.2). Scene survival following aortic trauma in road traffic accidents is reported to be less than 10% with an overall survival of only 2%.[19] However, endovascular techniques have now challenged the traditional surgical approach of thoracotomy and aortic replacement. Diagnosis of injury can be made by MDCT angiography, which has superseded contrast aortography as the imaging modality of choice. Anatomical suitability for thoracic endovascular aortic repair (TEVAR) can be confirmed by MDCT angiography from neck to pelvis. Such extensive imaging is necessary to confirm adequate size and morphology of the iliac arteries and distal aorta, (through which an endograft will have to be passed) and configuration of the aortic arch and its relationship to the site of aortic injury (which will determine graft size and the optimum site of deployment). Other important factors to take into consideration are patient stability, prioritization of coexistent injuries and the availability of a suitable endograft. Timing of repair remains a contentious issue. When faced with an uncomplicated (absence of pseudoaneurysm or rupture) dissection, medical management with careful blood pressure control and serial observation and imaging is appropriate. However, in the cases of complicated dissection with concurrent thoracic or extra-thoracic pathology, it may be justifiable to initially optimize the patient with careful blood pressure control and observation before considering definitive repair by open or endovascular means at a later stage. Recent data have confirmed that TEVAR can match open repair in terms of short- and medium-term outcome.[20] When this is combined with the minimally invasive nature of the technique, it is tempting to declare TEVAR as the superior treatment option. However, although meta-analysis of non randomized series suggests that early mortality and risk of paraplegia are lower with TEVAR, there is an absence of long-term follow-up data, let alone randomized data to compare TEVAR and open repair.[21] It seems unlikely that randomized trial data will be forthcoming, but as endograft technology improves and long-term, follow-up data accumulates, TEVAR will undoubtedly gain greater acceptance.

Injury to the abdominal aorta and visceral arteries represents a challenging problem and in-hospital mortality is reported to exceed 70%.[22] Typically, the injuries arise from penetrating rather than blunt trauma; diagnosis can be confirmed with MDCT. By contrast to the thoracic aorta, injuries of the visceral aorta are almost always managed with open surgical repair.[22] At present, endovascular technology is not far enough evolved to adequately tackle the branched aorta in an emergent setting. However, isolated injuries of the infra-renal aorta and iliac segment may be adequately managed using conventional abdominal aortic endografts. Once again, there is little high level evidence to support this practice, but the advantages of endovascular treatment are compelling when compared to open repair.

Key Point

- The use of thoracic stent grafts has led to a paradigm shift in the management of traumatic thoracic aortic dissection. However, uncertainty persists regarding long-term durability.

Pelvic Injury

Pelvic trauma with hemodynamic instability may be associated with a mortality rate of 18% to 40%.[23] Pelvic fractures may cause arterial, venous or fracture hematoma bleeding. More than 70% of unstable patients will have an associated arterial injury.[24] Such patients are generally injured in multiple sites and vulnerable to the sequelae of polytrauma and shock. Injury is again best assessed using MDCT. It has great utility in distinguishing venous from arterial injuries. Isolated pelvic bleeding in an unstable patient is now probably best managed by endovascular intervention. Orthopedic fixation of the unstable pelvis in a patient with hemodynamic compromise may be supported by temporary balloon occlusion of the internal iliac arteries. The most frequently injured arteries are the superior gluteal, internal pudendal, lateral sacral, iliolumbar and

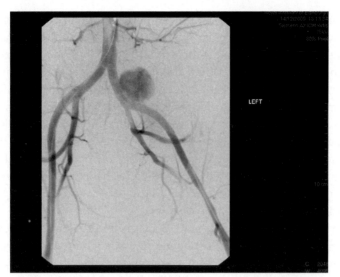

Fig. 13.3A: Digital subtraction angiogram of left common iliac artery false aneurysm caused by penetrating injury.

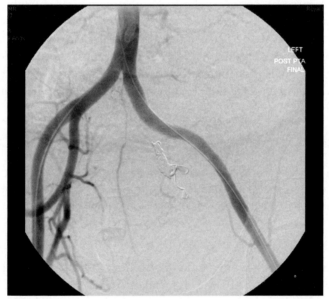

Fig. 13.3B: Digital subtraction angiogram of left common iliac artery false aneurysm excluded by internal iliac coil embolization and common iliac stenting.

inferior gluteal. Targeted endovascular embolization can be performed either selectively into the bleeding vessel or non-selectively, in particularly unstable patients, into the internal iliac or other feeding arterial stem (Figs 13.3A and B). In the rare scenario where a bleeding source cannot be clearly identified and the patient remains unstable, empirical bilateral internal iliac embolization may be performed. Embolic agents include absorbable gelatin sponge (gelfoam), which causes temporary arterial occlusion followed by eventual recanalization or coils, which cause permanent occlusion. Endovascular embolization of pelvic arterial bleeding may be successful in over 85% of cases.[25] Its use is associated with a far lesser mortality than open hemorrhage control but once again there are no randomized data to support its practice. Recently, the effectiveness of endovascular embolization has been called into question and there are data to support a strategy of routine external fixation and open preperitoneal pelvic packing in patients with hemodynamic instability and pelvic fracture.[23] Angiography and embolization is only used where there is a subsequent concern of ongoing blood loss. This approach is said to improve mortality rates compared to routine angiography and embolization.

Key Point

- The majority of vascular injuries will continue to require a traditional open surgical approach.

Extremity Injury

Vascular injury of the extremities may manifest as the classical cold white limb or with major hemorrhage. However, lesser injuries, such as intimal tears may elude diagnosis unless they are considered in the presence of an appropriate mechanism of injury, such as joint dislocation or long bone fracture. The brachial artery is the most commonly injured vessel in the body and is implicated in 20 to 30% of peripheral arterial injuries (Fig. 13.4).[26] Injury to the distal popliteal artery carries a high risk of limb loss, as the collateral circulation is not well developed around the knee.

Endovascular management of peripheral vascular injuries is seldom achievable and direct surgical exploration is usually required. This restriction is largely influenced by the diminishing caliber of peripheral arteries, their proximity to mobile joints and the uncertain long-term patency of endovascular grafts. However, there are some instances where covered stents or embolization techniques may be useful. Arteriovenous fistulae can be treated with covered stents and small pseudoaneurysms by percutaneous thrombin injection or embolization.

SUMMARY

Vascular trauma will continue to challenge surgeons. However, recent advances have armed surgeons with new strategies to investigate and treat such injured patients. The effectiveness and application of these measures is often dependent upon a cohesive, multidisciplinary approach involving a team of emergency medicine physicians, interventional radiologists, anesthetists and vascular surgeons. The relationship between hospital and surgeon volume and patient outcomes is increasingly recognized and it

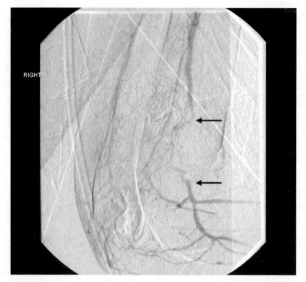

Fig. 13.4: Digital subtraction angiogram showing complete disruption of right brachial artery (black arrows) caused by fracture dislocation of elbow.

is important that patients are managed in centers with a contemporary infrastructure and appropriate levels of on-site expertise wherever possible. It is important to recognize that an endovascular solution in arterial injuries is achievable in around 10% of all cases treated. There is evidence to suggest that endovascular interventions are associated with shorter hospital stays and improved survival.[27]

REFERENCES

1. Gupta R, Rao S, Sieunarine K. An epidemiological view of vascular trauma in Western Australia: A 5-year study. ANZ J Surg 2001;71:461-6.
2. Bickell WH, Wall Jr MJ, Pepe PE, et al. Immediate versus delayed fluid resuscitation for hypotensive patients with penetrating torso injuries. N Engl J Med 1994;331:1105-9,
3. Dutton RP, Mackenzie CF, Scalea TM. Hypotensive resuscitation during active hemorrhage: impact on in-hospital mortality. J Trauma 2002;52: 1141-6.
4. Schreiber MA, Tieu B. Hemostasis in Operation Iraqi Freedom III. Surgery 2007;142:S61-6.
5. Todd SR, Malinoski D, Muller PJ, Schreiber MA. Hextend attenuates hypercoagulability after severe liver injury in swine. J Trauma 2005;59: 589-93.
6. Gan TJ, Bennett-Guerrero E, Phillips-Bute B, et al. Hextend, a physiologically balanced plasma expander for large volume use in major surgery: a randomized phase III clinical trial. Anesth Analg 1999;88:992-8.
7. Brohi K. Diagnosis and management of coagulopathy after major trauma. Br J Surg 2009;96:963-4.

8. Borgman MA, Spinella PC, Perkins JG, et al. The ratio of blood products transfused affects mortality in patients receiving massive transfusions at a combat support hospital. J Trauma 2007;63:805-13.

9. Snyder CW, Weinberg JA, McGwin G Jr, et al. The relationship of blood product ratio to mortality: survival benefit or survival bias? J Trauma 2009; 66:58-62.

10. Holcomb JB, Wade CE, Michalek JE, Chisholm GB, Zarzabal LA, Schreiber MA, et al. Increased plasma and platelet to red blood cell ratios improves outcome in 466 massively transfused civilian trauma patients. Ann Surg 2008;248:447-58.

11. Schreiber MA, Holcomb JB, Hedner U, Brundage SI, Macaitis JM, Hoots K. The effect of recombinant factor VIIa on coagulopathic pigs with grade V liver injuries. J Trauma 2002;53:252-7.

12. Friederich PW, Henny CP, Messelink EJ, et al. Effect of recombinant activated factor VII on perioperative blood loss in patients undergoing retropubic prostatectomy: a double-blind placebo-controlled randomised trial. Lancet 2003;361:201-5.

13. Boffard KD, Riou B Warren B, et al. Recombinant factor VIIa as adjunctive therapy for bleeding control in severely injured trauma patients: two parallel randomized, placebo-controlled, double-blind clinical trials. J Trauma 2005; 59:8-15.

14. Perkins J, Schreiber MA, Wade CE, Holcomb JB. Early vs late recombinant factor VIIa usage in trauma patients requiring massive transfusion in combat support hospitals. J Trauma 2006;61:505.

15. Schwartz MR, Weaver FA, Bauer M, Siegel A, Yellin AE. Refining the indications for arteriography in penetrating extremity trauma: a prospective analysis. J Vasc Surg 1993;17:116-22.

16. Seamon MJ, Smoger D, Torres DM, Pathak AS, Gaughan JP, Santora TA, et al. A prospective validation of a current practice: the detection of extremity vascular injury with CT angiography. J Trauma. 2009;67:238-4.

17. White PW, Gillespie DL, Feurstein I, et al. Sixty-Four Slice Multidetector Computed Tomographic Angiography in the Evaluation of Vascular Trauma. J Trauma 2010;68:96-102.

18. Tambyraja AL, Scollay JM, Beard D, Henry JM, Murie JA, Chalmers RT. Aortic trauma in Scotland—a population based study. Eur J Vasc Endovasc Surg 2006;32:686-9.

19. Richens D, Kotidis K, Neale M, Oakley C, Fails A. Rupture of the aorta following road traffic accidents in the United Kingdom 1992-1999. The results of the co-operative crash injury study. Eur J Cardiothorac Surg 2003; 23:143-8.

20. Xenos ES, Abedi NN, Davenport DL, Minion DJ, Hamdallah O, Sorial EE, et al. Meta-analysis of endovascular vs open repair for traumatic descending thoracic aortic rupture. J Vasc Surg 2008;48:1343-51.

21. Azizzadeh A, Keyhani K, Miller CC 3rd, Coogan SM, Safi HJ, Estrera AL. Blunt traumatic aortic injury: initial experience with endovascular repair. J Vasc Surg 2009;49:1403-8.

22. Deree J, Shenvi E, Fortlage D, et al. Patient factors and operating room resuscitation predict mortality in traumatic abdominal aortic injury: a 20-year analysis. J Vasc Surg 2007;45:493-7.

23. Cothren CC, Osborn PM, Moore EE, et al. Preperitoneal packing for hemodynamically unstable pelvic fractures: A paradigm shift. J Trauma 2007; 62:3834-42.

24. Anderson SW, Soto JA, Lucey BC, et al. Blunt trauma: Feasibility and clinical utility of pelvic CT angiography performed with 64-detector row CT, Radiology 2008;246:410-9.

25. Eastridge BJ, Starr A, Minei JP, et al., The importance of fracture pattern in guiding therapeutic decision-making in patients with hemorrhagic shock and pelvic ring disruptions. J Trauma 2002;53:446-50.

26. Mattox KL, Brundage SI, Hirshberg A. Vascular trauma. In: Townsend CM (Ed). Sabiston Textbook of Surgery: The Biological Basis of Modern Surgical Practice, WBSaunders, Philadelphia, PA 2001;1403-17.

27. Reuben BC, Whitten MG, Sarfati M, Kraiss LW. Increasing use of endovascular therapy in acute arterial injuries: analysis of the National Trauma Data Bank. J Vasc Surg 2007;46:1222-6.

SECTION SEVEN

RANDOMIZED TRIALS
IN SURGERY

CHAPTER FOURTEEN

Assessment of Randomized Controlled Trials in Surgery

Kurinchi S Gurusamy, Brian R Davidson

INTRODUCTION

The quality of the evidence, the importance of the outcomes and the degree to which a treatment affects an outcome ('effect') are the major factors that determine the recommendations of guideline developers with regards to the use of any individual treatment for a particular disease.[1] Evidence based on randomized controlled trials (RCTs) is considered the highest level or quality of evidence available for estimating the beneficial and harmful effects ('effect estimate') of an intervention.[1,2] However, a biased randomized controlled trial can downgrade the quality of evidence[1] and result in a decreased level of recommendation.

Bias is defined as 'predisposition towards' or 'prejudice' or 'systematic distortion'.[3] Bias in a RCT can be defined as the risk of predisposition towards either the experimental intervention group or the control group. Bias in RCTs may over or underestimate the true benefits and harms of an intervention (bias in 'effect estimate').[4-7] In other words, risk of bias can result in a deviation from the true effect estimate. An illustration of the effect of bias is shown in Figure 14.1. The word 'Effectiveness' is projected on a purple screen. The size of the word on the screen represents the magnitude of the effect observed in a particular study. Behind the screen (to the left of the screen in the figure), the actual word is shown in different scenarios of bias, such as underestimation, true estimation, overestimation and estimation in the wrong direction. In order to know whether the effect estimate obtained in the RCT is a true portrayal or a distorted portrayal (distorted in way of underestimation, overestimation or estimation in the wrong direction) of the true effect, it is necessary to assess bias and generalizability. The risk of bias in a trial is also known as 'internal validity' of the trial as opposed to 'external validity', which can be described as whether the study is designed appropriately to answer the research question.[8] Generalizability of a study can be described as the population in which the results can be used.

Key Point

- Bias in randomized controlled trials can result in incorrect assessment of the effectiveness of a treatment.

Various scales and checklists have been suggested for the assessment of risk of bias.[9,10] The current belief of experts in evidence-based medicine is that bias has to be estimated in various domains (components in trial design).[8] Recently, The Cochrane Handbook for Systematic Review of Interventions,[8] as well as the Cochrane Hepato-Biliary Group (CHBG) module, [11] which provides the guidelines for preparation of reviews registered with the CHBG were updated. Both sources recommend using various domains or components for the assessment of risk of bias. A summary of the various sources of bias that exist in the trials and the domains that assess these various sources of bias is shown in Table 14.1.

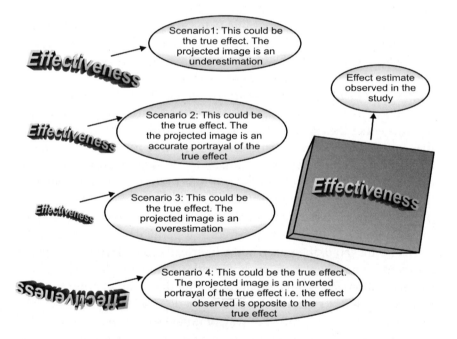

Fig. 14.1: Illustration of the effects of bias in study design. A word 'Effectiveness' is projected on a purple screen. The size of the word on the screen represents the magnitude of the effect observed in the study. Behind the screen (to the left of the screen in the figure), the actual word is shown in different scenarios. In scenario 1, the effect observed is an underestimation of the true effect. In scenario 2, the effect observed is a true portrayal of the true effect. In scenario 3, the effect is an overestimation of the true effect. In scenario 4, the effect observed is completely opposite to the true effect.

TABLE 14.1

Summary of domains and the bias related to each domain (modified from the Cochrane Handbook for Systematic Reviews of Interventions)[8]

Source of bias	Description	Domain assessed
Selection bias	Systematic differences between baseline characteristics of the groups that are compared	Randomization Baseline imbalance Source of funding
Performance bias	Systematic differences between groups in the care that is provided, or in exposure to factors other than the interventions of interest	Blinding Source of funding
Detection bias	Systematic differences between groups in how outcomes are determined	Blinding Source of funding
Attrition bias	Systematic differences between groups in withdrawals from a study	Incomplete data outcome Source of funding
Reporting bias	Systematic differences between reported and unreported findings	Selective outcome reporting Source of funding
Inappropriate outcome bias	Bias resulting from choosing an inappropriate surrogate or composite outcome	Selective outcome reporting
Early stopping bias	Trials are stopped at a point when the treatment effect is at random high when an insufficient number of outcome measures have been achieved	Early stopping Source of funding
Academic bias	A bias towards finding the same result if the clinical trial is repeated in a new group of patients	Academic bias
Source of funding bias	A bias towards finding results that favor additional income for the funder	Source of funding
Differential expertise bias	Bias resulting from systematic differences in the expertise of the health care provider in providing the intervention and control	Differential expertise bias

Key Point

- Different aspects of trial design (domains) can contribute to bias in a randomized controlled trial and each domain can be assessed individually.

The main domains of risk of bias assessment are randomization, blinding, incomplete data outcome bias, selective reporting bias, baseline imbalance bias, early stopping bias, academic bias and source of funding bias. Further details of these domains and biases and the methods that can be used to avoid these biases are explained in this review. Situations are also considered in which it is impossible or difficult to achieve low risk of bias in some components and the dilemma that a researcher faces during trial design to achieve low risk of bias in these components.

A variety of trial designs exists with different risks of bias. In parallel design trials, each participant is randomly allocated to intervention or control group. In cross-over randomized controlled trials, all the participants receive both treatments (intervention and control) in sequence with a 'wash-out' period between the two treatments in order to allow the effect of one treatment to stop. The order in which the treatment is performed is randomized. In cluster randomized controlled trial design, a group of patients are randomly allocated to intervention or control. All patients registered with a general practitioner allocated to intervention will receive the same interventional treatment. Patients visiting general practitioners allocated to control will all act as controls. Cross-over cluster randomized trials are also possible. Since the majority of surgical trials are of parallel trial design, only the guidelines pertaining to parallel trial design are discussed.

RANDOMIZATION PROCESS

The primary aim of randomization is to decrease selection bias (systematic differences between baseline characteristics of the groups that are compared)[8] i.e. to ensure that the same sort of participants receive each intervention. Randomization achieves this by making it impossible to predict whether a patient will receive the intervention or control. Take for example, a trial comparing palliative cytoreductive surgery (removal of as much tumor as feasible by surgical resection) versus other forms of palliative treatment for liver metastases from gastro-entero-pancreatic neuroendocrine tumors. Palliative cytoreductive surgery is generally performed only if 70 to 90% of the tumor can be resected or ablated.[12] If survival in patients who underwent palliative cytoreductive surgery was compared with survival in patients in whom palliative cytoreductive surgery could not be performed for reasons, such as the general condition of the patient or likelihood of not being able to remove at least 70% of tumor, factors other than the intervention could be responsible for any difference noted in survival. It would be wrong to attribute the improvement in survival to cytoreductive surgery. Such a bias resulting from selection of fundamentally different patients in different groups is common in the published surgical literature and is called selection bias. This bias is overcome by randomization.

The randomization process consists of two components 'generation of the allocation sequence' and 'allocation concealment'. Generation of allocation sequence corresponds to the development of a sequence or order in which the patients will be allocated to intervention or control. If future allocation of patient to intervention or control ('allocation') can be predicted because of improper sequence generation, such as alternation (patients alternately allocated to receive treatment A or treatment B), patients who may not be suitable for cytoreductive surgery because of inability to achieve 70 to 90% debulking may be enrolled into the trial if the next treatment option is not surgery. This method of improper sequence generation may result in a selection bias similar to the one that results if no randomization was used and may overestimate the survival benefit of cytoreductive surgery. Other improper methods of generation of allocation sequence include allocation by date of birth, allocation by hospital number, allocation by the day of the week or allocation by the date of hospital admission. Appropriate methods of generation of allocation sequence include the use of a random number table, computer-generated sequence, toss of coin or by shuffling.

Randomization can be achieved only if the allocation sequence generated by an appropriate method is concealed to the person who recruits the patient into the trial. An improper method of allocation concealment, such as use of an open allocation list (an open list, which contains the sequence in which the patients will be allocated to different treatments) can result in selection bias (and overestimate the survival benefit of treatment) as the recruiter is able to predict the group to which the next patient will be allocated. The commonly used methods for allocation concealment include the use of opaque, sequentially numbered, sealed envelopes or an allocation sequence held by a third party not involved in the recruitment of the patients.[8] Current recommendation is to avoid 'envelope' randomization (which can easily lead to violation of the allocation sequence).

Allocation concealment is commonly confused with 'blinding'. Blinding refers to the process by which study participants, personnel and outcome assessors are kept unaware of intervention allocations after inclusion and randomization of participants into the trial[11] in order to avoid performance bias (systematic differences between the groups in the care that is provided) and detection bias (systematic differences between the groups in how the outcomes are determined). It is possible to achieve adequate allocation concealment without blinding (as in the example palliative cytoreductive surgery versus other palliative treatments, where it is possible to allocate a patient to intervention or control randomly but once the allocation is done, it is not possible to perform the treatment (intervention or control) without the surgeon knowing what the treatment is. It is also not possible to perform the treatment (intervention or control) without the patient knowing what the allocation is. It is possible to achieve blinding with inadequate allocation concealment. For example, a study which compares pancreaticogastrostomy (PG) with pancreatico-jejunostomy (PJ) after pancreatoduodenectomy may allocate patients by hospital number. If the patients are not informed of the way the treatment was decided and what treatment was carried out, they will be blinded to the treatment groups.

There are two special situations in randomization. The first is the use of blocked randomization, which divides the sample required to complete the trial into different blocks (multiple samples of fewer number of participants) in order to ensure that participants are allocated in the desired ratio,[8] say 50% intervention and 50% control or 75% intervention and 25% control. For example, patients can be divided into blocks of four patients each. Among these four patients, two patients can be allocated to intervention and two patients can be allocated to control. However, if there is lack of blinding, it is possible to predict the future allocation with certainty in 25% to 50% of the patients of each block. Use of a larger block size and blocks of variable sizes decreases the ability to predict future allocation.

The second special situation is the 'minimization' process. Minimization has been suggested as an alternative to randomization.[13] In the minimization process, patients are allocated to the different groups by a third party (not involved in patient recruitment or subsequent patient care) depending upon the allocation of the previous patients with a view to balance the intervention and control groups for important prognostic factors.[13] This can work in multicenter trials with appropriate methods of blinding and can be considered to be equivalent to adequate randomization in decreasing selection bias.[8] However, in the presence of lack of blinding, particularly in a single center trial, it is easy to predict the next assignment if the method of minimization is known. This may introduce bias.

Key Point

- Randomization using appropriate techniques ensures that the same sort of participants receive each intervention and can be achieved in most trials in surgery.

BLINDING OF PARTICIPANTS, PERSONNEL AND OUTCOME ASSESSORS

The purpose of blinding is to decrease performance bias and detection bias.[11] For example, in a trial assessing the use of abdominal drains, if the surgeon knew that a drain would not be placed, he might take extra care in hemostasis than if he knew that a drain would be placed. This may indirectly benefit the 'no drainage' group, introducing performance bias.

Detection bias occurs when there is a lack of blinding of patients and outcome assessors. In a trial comparing laparoscopic liver resection and open liver resection, if the patient is aware that he/she has undergone laparoscopic liver resection, he/she may report less pain because that is what is expected to happen. A difference in the way questions are asked ("do you need pain relief?" or "don't you need pain relief?" carry different recommendations to the patient) or a comment ("I am surprised that you need so much pain relief!") may result in a change in outcomes. Thus, lack of observer blinding might introduce detection bias.

Use of placebos enables blinding of patients, health care providers and outcome observers in trials assessing pharmacological interventions. However, successful blinding of all three groups is difficult or impossible in surgical trials. Sham operations may be ideal in comparisons involving surgery. However, in practice, this is undesirable or even unethical due to the risks of the sham operation.

Blinding of the surgeon is obviously impossible in many surgical trials. However, blinding of surgeons can be achieved in some situations. In trials involving assessment of abdominal drainage in different surgeries, the drain can be placed by a second surgeon who is not otherwise involved in the surgery or assessment.

Blinding of outcome assessors is reported in less than half of surgical trials.[14] This is because the surgeon, who performed the surgery, is also often the outcome assessor. By involving another surgeon (not involved in the surgery and blinded to the treatment provided) in the postoperative assessment of the patient, it is possible to achieve assessor blinding. Other members of the team, such as nurses or research assistants can assess some outcomes that do not involve alteration of the management plan of the patient. Use of objective outcomes,[7] which cannot be easily influenced by the patient or the investigator (such as all-cause mortality, recognized laboratory tests,[7] use of universally accepted definitions for outcomes, clearly defining the outcomes, if no universal definition exists, pre-specified criteria for investigation and pre-specified criteria for treatment based on laboratory tests or radiological investigations interpreted by doctors blinded to the groups) can minimize the risk of bias due to lack of surgeon blinding.

Occasionally, it may not be possible to decrease bias due to the lack of blinding. Take for example, laparoscopic cholecystectomy versus no cholecystectomy for gallbladder dyskinesia. The main reason for cholecystectomy is the relief of symptoms. This is a subjective measure in a circumstance in which a sham operation would be the only way to achieve blinding of patients. Thus, one has to balance between the risks of providing treatment based on biased trials or a more complex trial design to obtain a result free from bias introduced by the lack of blinding.

INCOMPLETE OUTCOME DATA

The researchers conducting the trial should take adequate precautions against 'attrition bias' (systematic differences between groups because of withdrawals after randomization). Attrition bias increases if the reasons for exclusion are related to the treatment.[15] The simplest way to avoid this bias is to avoid post-randomization withdrawals (drop-outs). This is achievable in surgical trials where short-term outcomes are evaluated and the interval between randomization and treatment is short. Randomization should be timed properly. For example, in a trial assessing pancreatico-gastrostomy versus pancreaticojejunostomy after pancreaticoduo-denectomy for cancer of the head of the pancreas, the randomization should be performed during the operation but after ensuring that the pancreaticoduodenectomy is performed in order to avoid post-randomization drop-outs due to inoperability of the cancer. This will avoid bias due to incomplete outcome data.

In some situations, it is not possible to avoid post-randomization dropouts. In a trial assessing the use of perioperative somatostatin analogs for preventing pancreatic leaks following pancreatic resection, the first study dose may be given preoperatively[16] so the patients are randomized preoperatively. However, 8 to 33% of patients will have unresectable tumor at operation.[17] One is still able to assess the role of somatostatin analogues following pancreatic resection with low risk of bias due to incomplete outcome data (inspite of post-randomization drop outs). One can be certain that the use of somatostatin did not result in non-operability, i.e. it did not influence the post-randomization dropouts. However, it is necessary to report the outcomes in the intervention and control groups of patients who did not undergo pancreatic resection in order to ensure that the study drug did not cause any increase in the adverse effects in these patients. Situations like this are rare and trials with post-randomization dropouts should be considered to be at high risk of incomplete data outcome bias in most situations. For example, in a trial to assess the role of preoperative biliary drainage in jaundiced patients undergoing pancreatic resection for pancreatic cancer, delay before surgery because of the preoperative biliary drainage may contribute to inoperability. Excluding inoperable patients from survival outcomes may result in a significant bias favoring preoperative biliary drainage.

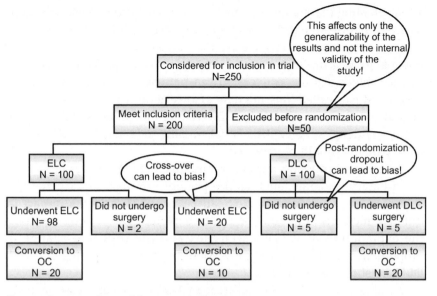

N = number or patients; OC = open cholecystectomy

Fig. 14.2: Patient flow: Early laparoscopic cholecystectomy (ELC)
versus delayed laparoscopic cholecystectomy (DLC).

The impact of post-randomization dropouts can be assessed using various methods of analysis. Consider a trial of laparoscopic cholecystectomy (LC) for patients with acute cholecystitis performed either early laparoscopic cholecystectomy (ELC) or delayed laparoscopic cholecystectomy (DLC). Hundred patients were allocated to each arm. Two patients allocated ELC refused surgery and 20 of the remaining 98 patients needed conversion to open cholecystectomy. Of the 100 patients in the DLC arm, 20 patients required early surgery because of non-resolution of symptoms or recurrence of symptoms and can be considered as 'crossovers'. Of these 20 patients, 10 patients required conversion to open cholecystectomy. Of the remaining 80 patients, five patients refused surgery after 6 weeks as their symptoms were resolved. Of the remaining 75 patients, 10 patients required conversion to open cholecystectomy. This is summarized in Figure 14.2.

The exclusion of patients before the randomization will affect the generalizability of the review but will not result in bias due to incomplete outcome data. Post-randomization dropouts and crossovers can result in a bias due to incomplete outcome data. The various methods of analysis that can be performed in this situation are 'intention-to-treat' analysis, 'available case analysis' ('complete case analysis'), 'per-protocol analysis' and 'treatment-received analysis'. In intention-to-treat analysis, all patients randomly allocated to one of the treatments in a trial are analyzed together as representing that treatment, whether or not they completed, or indeed received that treatment.[18] When there are post-randomization dropouts, it may not be possible to measure the outcomes. In this trial, it is not possible to measure the outcome 'conversion to open cholecystectomy' (simply referred to as 'conversion') in patients who did not undergo surgery. This is called 'missing data'. However, it is possible to measure the outcome 'pancreatitis' during the waiting time in these patients who did not undergo surgery. This is not missing data and the outcomes of these patients should be reported.

When data is missing, various imputation methods are applicable.[19,20] For a binary outcome, such as the presence or absence of benefit or complication, various scenarios can be applied[11] and the impact of different methods of imputation can be explored. The various scenarios, the explanation of various scenarios and the resulting change in proportions in each group for 'conversion' in the trial comparing ELC with DLC are shown in Table 14.2.

An alternative to intention-to-treat analysis is 'available case analysis' ('complete case analysis'). In available case analysis, data are analyzed for every participant for whom the outcome was obtained[8] and the patients are analyzed according to the group to which they were randomized. In the above example, an available case analysis may be more appropriate than the intention-to-treat analysis with imputation, if the aim was to assess the differences in complication rates. Two other analyses 'per-protocol analysis' (only participants who completed the trial and who received the allocated treatment are included in the analyses)[8] and 'treatment-received analysis' (participants are analyzed according to the interventions received irrespective of the allocation)[8] should be avoided in superiority trials (trials designed to identify superiority of one treatment over another). In the above example, patients belonging to the DLC group who required ELC because of non-resolution, worsening of symptoms or because of recurrence of symptoms during the waiting period had a high conversion rate. These patients will be excluded by following a 'per-protocol analysis'. Worse still, they will be included under ELC by 'treatment-received analysis'.

In trials, designed to investigate whether a treatment is therapeutically similar or not inferior to another treatment (equivalence and non-inferiority trials), per-protocol analysis may be better than intention-to-treat analysis in specific situations.[21] However, it is debatable whether equivalence or non-inferiority trials should be performed at all.[22]

Various methods of imputation are available to predict missing data for continuous outcomes, such as hospital stay.[23] Multiple imputation is one of the most reliable methods;[24] this can be performed using statistical software, such as STATA or SPSS.

TABLE 14.2

Different methods of analysis of a binary outcome in the presence of post-randomization dropouts and/or crossovers

Types of analysis	Description	Early laparoscopic chole-cystectomy (ELC) n/N (Percentage)	Delayed laparoscopic cholecystec-tomy (DLC) n/N (Percentage)	Statistical significance (Fisher's exact test)	Explanation
Intention-to-treat analysis (good outcome)	All patients allocated to a treatment are analyzed in that group irrespective of whether they received the treatment or not (intention-to-treat analysis). All patients with missing data are considered to have good outcomes in both groups.	20/100 (20%)	20/100 (20%)	P > 0.9999 (not significant)	The crossovers (20 patients in the DLC who required ELC) are analyzed with DLC. The post-randomization dropouts are considered not to have required conversion to open cholecystectomy ('conversion').
Intention-to-treat analysis (poor outcome)	All patients with missing data are considered to have poor outcomes in both groups.	22/100 (22%)	25/100 (25%)	P = 0.622 (not significant)	The crossovers (20 patients in the DLC who required ELC) are analyzed with DLC. The post-randomization-dropouts are considered to have required conversion.
Intention-to-treat analysis (best case for ELC)	All patients in the intervention group with missing data are considered to have good outcome and all the patients in the control group with the missing data are considered to have poor outcome.	20/100 (20%)	25/100 (25%)	P = 0.404 (not significant)	The crossovers (20 patients in the DLC who required ELC) are analyzed with DLC. The post-randomization dropouts in ELC are considered not to have required conversion, while the post-randomization dropouts in DLC are considered to have required conversion.

Contd...

Table contd...

Types of analysis	Description	Early laparo-scopic chole-cystectomy (ELC) n/N (Percentage)	Delayed laparoscopic cholecystec-tomy (DLC) n/N (Percentage)	Statistical significance (Fisher's exact test)	Explanation
Intention-to-treat analysis (worst case for ELC)	All patients in the intervention group with missing data are considered not to have developed the beneficial outcome and all the patients in the control group with missing data are considered to have developed the beneficial outcome.	22/100 (22%)	20/100 (20%)	P = 0.7326 (not significant)	The crossovers (20 patients in the DLC who required ELC) are analyzed with DLC. The post-randomization dropouts in ELC are considered to have required conversion, while the post-randomization dropouts in DLC are considered not to have required conversion.
Available case analysis	All patients in whom the outcome can be measured will be included and will be included in the group to which they were initially allocated irrespective of what they actually received.	20/98 (20.4%)	20/95 (21.1%)	P = 0.9295	The crossovers (20 patients in the DLC who required ELC) are analyzed with DLC. The post-randomization dropouts in both groups are excluded from the analysis.
Per-protocol analysis	Only participants who received the allocated treatment will be included in the analysis.	20/98 (20.4%)	10/75 (13.3%)	P = 0.314	The crossovers and the post-randomization dropouts are excluded from the analysis in both groups.
Treatment-received analysis	Participants are analyzed according to the interventions received irrespective of the allocation.	30/118 (25.4%)	10/75 (13.3%)	P = 0.098	The crossovers (20 patients in the DLC who required ELC) are analyzed with ELC. The post-randomization dropouts in both groups are excluded from the analysis.

n = Number with conversion to open cholecystectomy
N = Total number of patients included in comparison
The data for this table is shown in Figure 14.2.

SELECTIVE REPORTING

Selective reporting refers to the practice of reporting only on the statistically significant beneficial outcomes and excluding the statistically non-significant outcomes or the harm outcomes. It can also result from using surrogate outcomes (a substitute for the actual outcome), which has not been validated. For example, using plasma values of aspartate transaminase (AST) instead of the clinical outcome of liver failure may result in an intervention seeming effective even when there is no difference in the recovery of the patient in any way. It is not safe to assume that the authors did not measure actual clinical outcomes (liver failure, hospital stay or intensive therapy unit stay).

Selective reporting can lead to bias in the effect estimate (an incorrect assumption that a treatment is more effective or less effective than the true effectiveness). Selective reporting may be failure to report a particular outcome or could occur when incomplete details are reported, which prevents inclusion of the results in a meta-analysis.[8] Selective reporting can sometimes invalidate the results of a trial. For example, in a trial assessing the role of low pressure pneumoperitoneum versus standard pressure pneumoperitoneum for performing laparoscopic cholecystectomy, if details on patients who had conversion to open cholecystectomy are not reported in the low pressure group, one cannot be certain about the safety of low pressure pneumoperitoneum. Selective outcome reporting may overestimate intervention effects by up to 100%.[25]

BASELINE IMBALANCE

In order that an intervention can be assessed properly, the participants in the trial should be matched for important characteristics i.e. there should be a balance between the groups at the baseline. Baseline imbalance may be due to improper randomization methods[8] or simply due to the 'play of chance'. In large trials (say more than 400 patients[26]), the randomization process ensures that there is no baseline imbalance. However, in smaller trials, this may not be achieved.

An imbalance in the baseline characteristics may raise doubts about the effectiveness and the applicability of the intervention. For example, in a trial comparing survival after pylorus preserving or standard resection for pancreatic cancer, if there was a difference in the number of patients with portal vein involvement (which is generally considered to be an adverse prognostic factor), any difference in survival between the treatment groups may be due to either the treatment or the prognostic difference. Stratification or minimization[13] should be considered in trial design, to reduce baseline imbalance in important prognostic factors (including the experience of the surgeons). Statistical methods, such as regression analysis may have to be used to adjust for any baseline imbalance that arises in spite of stratification or minimization.

EARLY STOPPING

Early stopping of a trial may also result in bias in the effect estimate[27] particularly if the trial was stopped early because the data demonstrated a beneficial effect of the intervention. In the course of the trial, early results may favor the intervention and this may even out in the long run. However, early stopping of the trial (even with formal stopping rules) stops the trial when the observed effectiveness is the highest.[27] This may not be the true effect of the treatment. It is not possible to determine if recruitment to the trial was stopped early unless sample size calculations were reported in the trial.

ACADEMIC BIAS

It is common to perform a pilot trial before performing an appropriately powered trial. If the researcher found interesting results in a pilot trial but does not find similar results in a larger randomized clinical trial, there may be a temptation to look for positive results using multiple statistical or subgroup analyses. Publication of the protocol in a trials register,[28] before the trial starts (e.g., at www.clinicaltrials.gov) will help in the assessment of this bias. Mandatory explanation of any deviation from the protocol might lead to a reduction in academic bias.

SOURCE OF FUNDING

A bias in the effect estimate or in the interpretation of the data[29,30] favoring additional income to the funder can result if the trial is funded by a party with vested interest in the success of the intervention. Other biases, such as 'early stopping bias', 'selective reporting bias', inappropriate comparator treatment and lack of peer reviewed publication of results are other possible reasons for source of funding bias.[30] Publication of the trial protocol should help in the identification of this bias.[28] By comparing the trial report with the protocol, it is possible to determine whether early stopping or selective reporting bias exists. The other domains (such as sequence generation, allocation concealment, blinding, missing outcomes and baseline imbalance) may also give a clue to the validity of such a trial.

DIFFERENTIAL EXPERTISE

A bias in the effect estimate can result if there are differences in the expertise of the health care provider in providing the intervention and control.[31] This can be either in the form of imbalance in the proportion of procedures performed by experienced and relatively inexperienced surgeons in the intervention and control arms or when a surgeon is more experienced in the control procedure than the intervention.

In the trial comparing ELC versus DLC for acute cholecystitis, if experienced surgeons perform ELC and relatively inexperienced surgeons perform DLC, a lower complication rate in ELC may result but this may be due to the difference in the experience of the surgeon and not due to the timing of surgery. This type of bias is a type of baseline imbalance bias. Stratification for surgical experience when there is a major difference in the experience of surgeons is required to avoid this bias.

In a trial comparing robotic assistant versus human assistant for laparoscopic cholecystectomy, if the surgeons do not have sufficient experience with using robotic assistant before the beginning of the trial, differences in instrument set-up time can be because of lack of previous experience in setting up the robotic assistant rather than because of true effect.[32]

Key Point

- The use of unvalidated surrogate outcomes, imbalance in the baseline characteristics of prognostic significance, early stopping of trials without formal stopping rules, conduct of trials by parties with vested interests (academic or industrial partner) and differences in the expertise of the health-provider in providing the intervention and control can all result in incorrect assessment of the effectiveness of a treatment.

CONCLUSION

Various guidelines exist for the conduct and reporting of randomized clinical trials.[33-39] Lack of adherence to such guidelines should alert the surgeon to the possibility of bias in the effect estimate. Careful assessment of the trials using an established framework for assessment of risk of bias (such as that used by the Cochrane collaboration) can lead to a better critical appraisal of randomized controlled trials and a better understanding of the utility of new interventions. This may also help surgeons to design and interpret the trial appropriately.

Key Point

- Better understanding of the sources of bias in randomized controlled trials can help in better study design and interpretation of results.

REFERENCES

1. Guyatt GH, Oxman AD, Kunz R, Vist GE, Falck-Ytter Y, Schunemann HJ, et al. What is "quality of evidence" and why is it important to clinicians? BMJ 2008;336(7651):995-8.
2. Harbour R, Miller J. A new system for grading recommendations in evidence based guidelines. BMJ 2001;323(7308):334-6.
3. Agarval B, Reddy AV, Labundy JL, Krishna NB. Ultrasonographic differential diagnosis of gallbladder polyps. Gastrointestinal Endoscopy 2008;67(5):AB213.
4. Kjaergard LL, Villumsen J, Gluud C. Reported methodologic quality and discrepancies between large and small randomized trials in meta-analyses. Ann Intern Med 2001;135(11):982-9.
5. Moher D, Pham B, Jones A, Cook DJ, Jadad AR, Moher M, et al. Does quality of reports of randomised trials affect estimates of intervention efficacy reported in meta-analyses? Lancet 1998;352(9128):609-13.
6. Schulz KF, Chalmers I, Hayes RJ, Altman DG. Empirical evidence of bias. Dimensions of methodological quality associated with estimates of treatment effects in controlled trials. JAMA 1995;273(5):408-12.
7. Wood L, Egger M, Gluud LL, Schulz KF, Juni P, Altman DG, et al. Empirical evidence of bias in treatment effect estimates in controlled trials with different interventions and outcomes: meta-epidemiological study. BMJ 2008;336(7644):601-5.
8. Higgins JPT, Green S, (editors). Cochrane Handbook for Systematic Reviews of Interventions Version 5.0.0 [updated February 2008]. The Cochrane Collaboration, 2008. Available at: wwwcochrane-handbookorg Accessed September 07, 2008.
9. Jadad AR, Moore RA, Carroll D, Jenkinson C, Reynolds DJ, Gavaghan DJ, et al. Assessing the quality of reports of randomized clinical trials: is blinding necessary? Control Clin Trials 1996;17(1):1-12.
10. Moher D, Jadad AR, Nichol G, Penman M, Tugwell P, Walsh S. Assessing the quality of randomized controlled trials: an annotated bibliography of scales and checklists. Control Clin Trials 1995;16(1):62-73.
11. Gluud C, Nikolova D, Klingenberg S, Alexakis N, Als-Nielsen B, D'Amico G, et al. The Cochrane Hepato-Biliary Group. About The Cochrane Collaboration (Cochrane Review Groups (CRGs)) 2008, Issue 4. Art. No.: LIVER. .
12. Chung MH, Pisegna J, Spirt M, Giuliano AE, Ye W, Ramming KP, et al. Hepatic cytoreduction followed by a novel long-acting somatostatin analog: a paradigm for intractable neuroendocrine tumors metastatic to the liver. Surgery 2001;130(6):954-62.
13. Scott NW, McPherson GC, Ramsay CR, Campbell MK. The method of minimization for allocation to clinical trials. a review. Control Clin Trials 2002;23(6):662-74.
14. Hall JC, Mills B, Nguyen H, Hall JL. Methodologic standards in surgical trials. Surgery 1996;119(4):466-72.
15. Tierney JF, Stewart LA. Investigating patient exclusion bias in meta-analysis. Int J Epidemiol 2005;34(1):79-87.
16. Sarr MG. The potent somatostatin analogue vapreotide does not decrease pancreas-specific complications after elective pancreatectomy: a prospective,

multicenter, double-blinded, randomized, placebo-controlled trial. Journal of the American College of Surgeons 2003;196(4):556-65.

17. Mayo SC, Austin DF, Sheppard BC, Mori M, Shipley DK, Billingsley KG. Evolving preoperative evaluation of patients with pancreatic cancer: does laparoscopy have a role in the current era? J Am Coll Surg 2009;208(1):87-95.

18. Newell DJ. Intention-to-treat analysis: implications for quantitative and qualitative research. Int J Epidemiol 1992;21(5):837-41.

19. Higgins JP, White IR, Wood AM. Imputation methods for missing outcome data in meta-analysis of clinical trials. Clin Trials 2008;5(3):225-39.

20. Hollis S, Campbell F. What is meant by intention to treat analysis? Survey of published randomised controlled trials. BMJ 1999;319(7211):670-4.

21. Matilde Sanchez M, Chen X. Choosing the analysis population in non-inferiority studies: per protocol or intent-to-treat. Stat Med 2006;25(7):1169-81.

22. Garattini S, Bertele V. Non-inferiority trials are unethical because they disregard patients' interests. Lancet 2007;370(9602):1875-7.

23. Wood AM, White IR, Thompson SG. Are missing outcome data adequately handled? A review of published randomized controlled trials in major medical journals. Clin Trials 2004;1(4):368-76.

24. Donders ART, van der Heijden GJMG, Stijnen T, Moons KGM. Review: A gentle introduction to imputation of missing values. J Clin Epidemiol 2006;59(10):1087-91.

25. Furukawa TA, Watanabe N, Omori IM, Montori VM, Guyatt GH. Association between unreported outcomes and effect size estimates in Cochrane meta-analyses. JAMA 2007;297(5):468-70.

26. Kernan WN, Viscoli CM, Makuch RW, Brass LM, Horwitz RI. Stratified randomization for clinical trials. J Clin Epidemiol 1999;52(1):19-26.

27. Bassler D, Montori VM, Briel M, Glasziou P, Guyatt G. Early stopping of randomized clinical trials for overt efficacy is problematic. J Clin Epidemiol 2008;61(3):241-6.

28. Wille-Jorgensen P, Gluud C. Prospective registration of clinical trials. Colorectal Dis 2006;8(1):1.

29. Als-Nielsen B, Chen W, Gluud C, Kjaergard LL. Association of funding and conclusions in randomized drug trials: a reflection of treatment effect or adverse events? JAMA 2003;290(7):921-8.

30. Lexchin J, Bero LA, Djulbegovic B, Clark O. Pharmaceutical industry sponsorship and research outcome and quality: systematic review. BMJ 2003;326(7400):1167-70.

31. Devereaux PJ, Bhandari M, Clarke M, Montori VM, Cook DJ, Yusuf S, et al. Need for expertise based randomised controlled trials. BMJ 2005; 330(7482):88.

32. Gurusamy KS, Samraj K, Fusai G, Davidson BR. Robot assistant for laparoscopic cholecystectomy. Cochrane Database Syst Rev 2009(1):CD006578.

33. Boutron I, Moher D, Altman DG, Schulz KF, Ravaud P. Methods and processes of the CONSORT Group: example of an extension for trials assessing nonpharmacologic treatments. Ann Intern Med 2008;148(4):W60-6.

34. Boutron I, Moher D, Altman DG, Schulz KF, Ravaud P. Extending the CONSORT statement to randomized trials of nonpharmacologic treatment: explanation and elaboration. Ann Intern Med 2008;148(4):295-309.

35. Gagnier JJ, Boon H, Rochon P, Moher D, Barnes J, Bombardier C. Reporting randomized, controlled trials of herbal interventions: an elaborated CONSORT statement. Ann Intern Med 2006;144(5):364-7.

36. Hopewell S, Clarke M, Moher D, Wager E, Middleton P, Altman DG, et al. CONSORT for Reporting Randomized Controlled Trials in Journal and Conference Abstracts: Explanation and Elaboration. PLoS Medicine 2008;5(1):e20.

37. Ioannidis JP, Evans SJ, Gotzsche PC, O'Neill RT, Altman DG, Schulz K, et al. Better reporting of harms in randomized trials: an extension of the CONSORT statement. Ann Intern Med 2004;141(10):781-8.

38. Moher D, Schulz KF, Altman D. The CONSORT statement: revised recommendations for improving the quality of reports of parallel-group randomized trials. JAMA 2001;285(15):1987-91.

39. Piaggio G, Elbourne DR, Altman DG, Pocock SJ, Evans SJ. Reporting of noninferiority and equivalence randomized trials: an extension of the CONSORT statement. JAMA 2006;295(10):1152-60.

CHAPTER FIFTEEN

Randomized Clinical Trials and Meta-analyses in Surgery 2009

Joanna Franks, Irving Taylor

Across all specialities, clinical practice is increasingly relying on a robust evidence base to support patient management. Surgery is no exception to this trend. This chapter highlights a selection of the randomized clinical trials and meta-analyses related surgery, which have been published in 2009.

GENERAL

Hospital acquired infections have recently featured in publications ranging from scientific journals to the popular press. In addition, it is a popular topic discussed in patient forums. A randomized controlled trial compared to commonly used forms of antiseptic, povidone iodine and 4% chlorhexidine,[1] to study the efficacy of the reduction of bacterial colonization and surgical wound infection. Five hundred patients aged 18-60 years undergoing surgery classified as clean, clean contaminated or contaminated were randomly divided into two groups and received one of the two skin preparations. Chlorhexidine 4% showed a significant reduction in bacterial colonization (14.4% vs 31.2%) and postoperative surgical wound infection (relative risk 1.61) and should be the first consideration for preoperative skin preparation.

Key Point

- Wound infection rates are reduced when 4% chlorhexidine is used to prepare the skin preoperatively.

Surgical site infection can result in many well documented sequelae, including wound breakdown. In recent years, vacuum dressings have gained popularity in managing this unfortunate complication, however, the dressing changes are painful. A double blind randomized prospective study was performed on 70 patients undergoing vacuum-assisted closure dressing changes to determine if 0.2% lidocaine administered through the tubing into the foam dressing 30 minutes before the change of dressing decreased the pain.[2] The control arm of the trial received 0.9% saline. Pain was assessed according to a 0-10 numeric pain scale. Patients who received lidocaine reported less pain than control patients both during the dressing change, 4.3 vs 6.3 (p = 0.005) and immediately after, 2.4 vs 4.7 (*p* = 0.001) respectively. The improved patient comfort during vacuum-assisted closure therapy achieved by the topical application of lidocaine may increase the number of patients who can successfully be managed in the community.

Key Point

• Topical administration of lidocaine prior to changing vacuum-assisted closure dressing improves patient comfort.

The management of cutaneous abscesses is usually undertaken by the on-call general surgeon. Standard treatment includes incision and drainage followed by packing. In a prospective, randomized single-blinded trial 48 patients with simple cutaneous abscesses, less than 5 cm in largest diameter were randomized to packing or no packing.[3] Patients treated with packing reported higher visual analog pain scores both at the time of the intervention (P = 0.014) and 48 hours after the procedure (*p* = 0.03), as well as greater use of analgesics. There was no significant difference in the need for a second intervention in the group who were managed without packing.

Key Point

• Simple cutaneous abscesses can be managed by incision and drainage followed by simple dressings without any increase in morbidity.

The placement of nasogastric (NG) tubes in surgical patients is common. Indications include decompression of the gastrointestinal tract, such as during the management of acute gastrointestinal obstruction, protection of anastomoses and increasingly for enteral feeding. Routine use of a NG tube has also been suggested to prevent postoperative nausea and vomiting. The data to support this hypothesis are however conflicting. A recent report compared patients with intraoperative or perioperative NG tubes to those without.[4] The incidence of postoperative nausea and vomiting in the operative NG tube group was 44.4% as compared with 41.5% in the control group (*p* = 0.35). In the perioperative NG tube group the incidence was 27.8% vs 31.3% in the control group.

The recognized indications for NG placement often require the procedure to be performed once the patient is anesthetized. It is however often difficult to place a NG tube correctly in this setting. A randomized controlled trial enrolled 200 patients into a study to determine which insertion technique would improve the success rate.[5] The simple modification of head flexion with lateral neck pressure was the easiest technique with the highest success rate and the fewest complications.

Key Point

- The incidence of postoperative nausea and vomiting is not reduced by the placement of an NG tube.

INCISIONAL HERNIA

Incisional hernias are commonly underestimated but probably complicate between 2 and 20% of all abdominal wall closures. Factors which affect incisional hernia rates can be divided into those relating to the surgery and those which are attributable to the individual patient. A recently published randomized controlled trial compared 150 patients who underwent a cholecystectomy and were randomly allocated to either a midline or transverse incision. The results demonstrated that after a minimum of 12 months follow-up, the incisional hernia rates were 2 and 14% for transverse and midline incisions respectively ($p = 0.017$). In addition, transverse incisions were found to be shorter and associated with a more pleasing appearance.[6]

Key point

- Transverse incisions result in fewer incisional hernias and should be considered in acute and elective open surgery of the upper abdomen.

The frequency of incisional hernias has resulted in a number of small randomized controlled trials comparing open and laparoscopic repair with mesh. A meta-analysis has been produced, which compared these two techniques and included data on effectiveness and safety.[7] Eight studies met the inclusion criteria. The results do not demonstrate any difference in hernia recurrence rates (relative risk 1.02). However, duration of hospital stay varied and the mean longest stay in the laparoscopic group was 5.7 days as compared with 10 days for open surgery. Laparoscopic surgery was also associated with fewer wound infections (relative risk 0.22) and a trend towards fewer hemorrhagic complications and infections requiring mesh removal.

Key point

- Laparoscopic incisional hernia repair is at least as effective as open repair and is associated with a shorter hospital stay and fewer complications.

UPPER GASTROINTESTINAL

Peptic Ulcer Disease

Increasing numbers of patients are regularly taking low dose aspirin as part of the management of cardiac or vascular disease. Few therapeutic options are available for the prevention of gastrointestinal mucosal damage. FAMOUS[8] is a recently published randomized double bind placebo controlled trial, which compared the protective affect of famotidine (20 mg BD), a well-tolerated histamine H_2-receptor antagonist, to placebo in patients taking between 75 mg and 325 mg of aspirin per day. At 12 weeks, 3.4% of the famotidine—treated patients had developed an ulcer on endoscopy compared with 15% in the placebo group (odds ratio 0.20). Only 0.5% of the famotidine treated patients had a duodenal ulcer and 4.4% had erosive esophagitis compared with 8.5 and 19% in the placebo group respectively.

Key Point

- Famotidine is effective in the prevention of gastric and duodenal ulcers and erosive esophagitis in patients taking low dose aspirin.

The main complications of peptic ulcer disease are bleeding and perforation. The management of both of these complications has been the subject of recent trials. The first line management of bleeding peptic ulcers is resuscitation and stabilization followed, in most hospitals, with an endoscopy aiming to control hemostasis. Ongoing active management includes proton pump inhibitors, which maintain intragastric pH at a neutral level and are therefore believed to reduce the rate of recurrent bleeding. A recent trial has evaluated the effect of various proton pump inhibitors given by different routes. Ninety consecutive patients with successful endoscopic therapy for a bleeding peptic ulcer underwent 72 hours of continuous ambulatory pH monitoring and were treated with either oral or IV preparations of omeprazole, pantoprazole and rabeprazole. There was no statistical difference between any of the proton pump inhibitors, all of which maintained a pH at between 6.11 and 6.93 compared with a mean pH of 2.04 in the control group. The route of administration did not affect the efficacy of the drugs.[9]

Key Point

- Proton pump inhibitors given orally or intravenously maintain a neutral intragastric pH and can be used to reduce the rate of recurrent peptic ulcer bleeding.

Laparoscopic surgery has become widely established in the elective surgical setting. Its benefit in emergency surgery is still the subject of clinical trials. A multicenter randomized clinical trial has been published, which evaluated whether laparorscopic closure of perforated peptic ulcer is as safe as the open surgical approach.[10] The postoperative visual analog pain scores were significantly lower in the laparoscopic patients (p < 0.05) on days 1, 3 and 7. Operating time in the laparoscopic patients was however longer, 75 vs 50 minutes, with comparable lengths of hospital stay in the two groups. Complications were equally distributed.

Key Point

- Laparoscopic repair of perforated peptic ulcer is a safe procedure with lower postoperative pain than open surgery.

Barrett's Esophagus

Barrett's esophagus is a condition characterized by intestinal metaplasia of the esophageal mucosa. It is associated with an increased risk of esophageal adenocarcinoma. A trial was conducted to determine whether endoscopic radiofrequency ablation could eradicate dysplastic Barratt's esophagus and decrease the rate of neoplastic progression.[11] Twelve months after treatment with radiofrequency ablation complete eradication of dysplasia occurred in 90.5% of low grade dysplasia patients and 81% of high grade dysplasia patients compared to 22.7 and 19% of the control groups respectively ($p < 0.001$). Patients in the ablation group had less disease progression (3.6% vs 16.3%) and fewer cancers (1.2% vs 9.3%). However, the treatment group did report more postprocedure chest pain, one patient (1.2%) had an upper gastrointestinal bleed and five patients (6%) developed an esophageal stricture.

Key Point

- Radiofrequency ablation of dysplastic Barrett's esophagus is associated with a high rate of complete eradication of both dysplasia and intestinal metaplasia and a reduced risk of disease progression.

Pyloric Stenosis

The management of infantile pyloric stenosis remains pyloromyotomy, however, a laparoscopic approach has gained popularity. The effectiveness of this approach remained unproven and the outcomes after open and laparoscopic pyloromyotomy have recently been the subject of a multicenter international randomized controlled trial in six tertiary pediatric centers.[12] Median time to achieve full enteral feeding in the laparoscopic group was 18.5 hours compared to 23.4 hours in the open group (p = 0.002). The average postoperative stay was shorter in the laparoscopic group (33.6 hours compared to 43.8 hours in the open patients). Intra- and postoperative complications, including vomiting were similar in the two groups. This trial was halted prior to full recruitment because of the significant benefit seen in the laparoscopic group on interim analysis of the data.

Key Point

- Laparoscopic pyloromyotomy is a safe procedure for the management of pyloric stenosis.

Esophageal Varices

The optimal management of esophagogastric varices is important because of their tendency to bleed with considerable morbidity, as well as high mortality. Varices have been the subject of several randomized trials published in 2009.

Octreotide and terlipressin are both established pharmacological therapies used in the management of variceal bleeding. One study[13] compared the efficacy and safety of these two drugs as an adjunct therapy to endoscopic variceal ligation in patients with esophageal variceal bleeding. Control of variceal bleeding was noted in 92.6% of patients treated with terlipressin where an average of 3.7 units of packed cells were required. In the octreotide group, 95.6% of patients had their bleeding controlled with an average transfusion of 3.9 units of packed cells. The length of hospital stay was significantly shorter for the terlipressin group, being on average 108 hours compared to 126 hours ($p \leq 0.001$) for the octreotide group. Terlipressin has the additional advantage of being effective in small intravenous bolus doses administered 4 hourly.

Key Point

- Terlipressin is an effective adjunct therapy for the control of esophageal variceal bleeding.

Endoscopic sclerotherapy is an established management strategy for acutely bleeding esophageal varices in cirrhotic patients. Emergency portocaval shunts are usually reserved as a second line treatment option. A randomized trial[14] compared these two treatment modalities in 211 unselected consecutive patients with cirrhosis and acutely bleeding esophageal varices who required at least two units of blood. Endoscopic sclerotherapy achieved permanent control of bleeding in 20% of patients compared to 100% of patients in the portocaval shunt group ($p \leq 0.001$). Compared with endoscopic sclerotherapy the patients in the portocaval shunt group had significantly higher survival ($p \leq 0.001$) across all Child's classes with a reduction in recurrent episodes of portal-systemic encephalopathy ($p \leq 0.01$).

> ## Key Point
>
> • Emergency portocaval shunts permanently stop variceal bleeding in cirrhotic patients and result in greater long-term survival and fewer complications.

A consequence of the portal hypertension seen in cirrhotic patients is hypersplenism. This complication is traditionally treated by splenectomy. However, this may be a hazardous operation in a patient with poor liver function. Angiographic advances have resulted in the increasing use of partial splenic embolization. A randomized trial[15] compared this new technique with splenectomy. In this study, partial splenic ligation was achieved using polyvinyl alcohol particles to achieve embolization in at least 50% of the distal branches of the splenic artery. All patients showed a marked improvement in both platelet and leukocyte counts. One patient in the embolization group (5%) developed a portal vein thrombosis compared to three patients (15%) in the splenectomy group. In addition, one patient in the embolization group developed splenic abscesses treated by a subsequent splenectomy. Partial splenic embolization was shown to be an effective therapeutic modality, which was safe and rapid to perform. It also has the additional benefit of allowing preservation of adequate splenic tissues to reduce the chance of overwhelming infection.

> ## Key Point
>
> • Partial splenic embolization is a rapid, safe and well-tolerated local anesthetic procedure, which can be used in the treatment of hypersplenism associated with cirrhosis.

HEPATO-PANCREATIC AND BILIARY

Hepatic Surgery

The management of colorectal liver metastasis requires accurate selection of patients who may benefit from surgical treatment. A randomized controlled trial of patients with colorectal liver metastasis investigated whether the addition of 18F-Fluoro-deoxyglucose positron emission tomography (18F-FDG PET) to conventional staging leads to improved clinical management and a reduction in futile laparotomies.[16] 150 patients with colorectal metastasis selected for surgical treatment by imaging with computed tomography (CT) were randomly assigned to CT only or CT plus 18F-FDG PET. Patient and tumor characteristics were similar in both groups. The number of laparotomies, which did not result in a disease free survival period longer than 6 months, was 45% in the control group and 28% in the experimental arm with 18F-FDG PET, corresponding to a risk reduction of 38%. ($p = 0.042$).

> **Key Point**
>
> - The addition of 18F-FDG PET to the work up for surgical resection of colorectal liver metastases prevents unnecessary surgery in 1 in 6 patients.

Pancreatic Surgery

Pancreatic fistula and intra-abdominal fluid collections are the commonest complications after distal pancreatectomy. Different techniques have been described all of which aim to reduce these complications and achieve perfect closure of the stump. A randomized controlled trial has compared the stapler technique with stapling combined with a seromuscular patch.[17] The overall rate of postoperative fistula or intra-abdominal fluid collection was higher in the stapling alone group. However, rates of clinically relevant postoperative complications, grade B or C fistula or fluid collection requiring treatment were comparable. The re-intervention rate and median hospital stay were similar in both groups.

> **Key Point**
>
> - Following distal pancreatectomy, covering the stapled pancreatic remnant with a seromuscular patch decreases overall pancreas- related complication, such as fistula.

Pancreatic cancer is renowned for its late presentation. The increased use of CT may result in an increase in the number of patients diagnosed with previously occult pancreatic carcinomas. A recently published randomized trial looked at whether adjuvant chemotherapy with gemcitabine improves the outcome of patients who have undergone a macroscopically curative resection of invasive ductal carcinoma of the pancreas.[18] Patients in the gemcitabine group showed significantly longer disease free survival with a recorded median of 11 months, compared with patients who were treated with surgery alone, who had a median survival of five months (hazard ratio = 0.60). However, the overall survival of the two groups did not differ significantly.

> **Key Point**
>
> - Adjuvant gemcitabine contributes to disease-free survival in patients undergoing macroscopically curative resection of the pancreas.

Biliary

Endoscopic retrograde cholangiography (ERCP) is firmly established in the management of gallstone disease. Its wide availability has resulted in increased research into preventing its well recognized complications.

One strategy, which has been adopted, is to improve pre-ERCP imaging. This would allow patients to be more accurately selected thereby reducing the number of procedures, which are performed. Endoscopic ultrasound (EUS) has emerged as an accurate diagnostic tool in the management of patients with choledocholithiasis. A systematic review of randomized controlled trials of EUS-guided ERCP vs ERCP in patients with suspected choledocholithiasis selected four eligible trials containing 213 patients.[19] In the EUS-guided ERCP group, ERCP was avoided in 67.1% of patients, resulting in a significant reduction in the overall risk of complications (relative risk 0.35, 95% confidence interval: 0.20-0.62) and post-ERCP pancreatitis (relative risk 0.21, 95% confidence interval: 0.06-0.83). Application of EUS, where available, in the selection of patients for therapeutic ERCP therefore, significantly reduces the complication rate.

Key Point

- Performing EUS, first in patients with suspected choledocholithiasis safely allows ERCP to be avoided in two-thirds of patients.

Altering the method by which an ERCP is performed, is an alternative way of reducing complications. A meta-analysis of randomized double-blind placebo-controlled trials has looked at whether prophylactic glyceryl trinitrate (GTN) treatment reduces the incidence of pancreatitis after ERCP.[20] Eight trials involving 1,920 patients were considered eligible for this study. Meta-analysis showed that the incidence of pancreatitis was 5.9% in the GTN group compared with 9.8% in the placebo group (P = 0.002). Patients who received GTN were 39% less likely to develop pancreatitis. Subgroup analysis suggested that the sublingual or transdermal route may be useful.

Key Point

- Post-ERCP complications, in particular pancreatitis, may be avoided by the routine use of GTN prior to the start of the procedure.

The technique used to cannulate the biliary tree has also been the subject of a meta-analysis.[21] Five randomized controlled trials were identified, which compared the standard contrast-assisted method with a wire-guided cannulation technique. The analysis of the primary cannulation rates of all the selected studies demonstrated that wire-guided cannulation yielded an odds ratio for success of 2.05 (95% confidence interval: 1.27-3.31). Comparing pancreatitis rates after wire-guided cannulation with those of the standard-method group yielded an odds ratio of 0.23 (95% confidence interval: 0.13-0.41). Although the results suggest that the wire-guided technique increases primary cannulation rates and reduces post-ERCP pancreatitis, further large randomized controlled trials are advised before this method is brought into mainstream practice.

Key Point

- Alteration of the technique to cannulate the biliary ducts with adoption of a wire-guided method increases the rate of cannulation, as well as reduces the incidence of pancreatitis after ERCP.

BARIATRIC SURGERY

Improvements in laparoscopic techniques along with the increase in the average BMI of Western populations have resulted in more research into this area. The surgery can be divided into procedures, which restrict intake and those which affect absorption.

Intake restriction can be achieved in several ways; a randomized study compared laparoscopic adjustable silicone gastric banding with laparoscopic vertical banded gastroplasty in morbid obesity.[22] One hundred patients with a BMI of 40-50 kg/m^2 were randomized to either technique and followed up for seven years. Late complication rates were 36.7% in the adjustable silicone gastric banding group compared with 15.7% in the vertical banded gastroplasty patients (p = <0.05) at 3 years. At five and seven years, the complication rate remained more favorable in the vertical banded gastroplasty group but the difference was not statistically significant. Late operation rates were significantly lower in the vertical banded gastroplasty group during the follow-up period, at year seven, it was 7.8% compared to 46.9% (p = <0.001) in the adjustable silicone gastric banding group. In addition, the excess weight loss was consistently greater in the vertical-banded gastroplasty patients.

Key Point

- In carefully selected morbidly obese patients laparoscopic vertical-banded gastroplasty results in significantly more weight loss than laparoscopic adjustable silicone gastric banding.

The indications for bariatric surgery vary depending on an individual's BMI and the presence of serious co-existing medical conditions, such as diabetes. The exclusion of the proximal small intestine is thought to play a major role in the rapid improvement in the metabolic control of glucose achieved by gastric bypass. A randomized prospective study has compared the effects of laparoscopic Roux-en-Y gastric bypass with laparoscopic sleeve gastrectomy on fasting and meal-stimulated insulin, glucose and glucagon-like peptide levels.[23] Excess BMI loss was similar for three months after both procedures. After surgery each group of patients had markedly increased postprandial plasma insulin and glycagon-like peptide levels (p = <0.01) both of which favor improved glucose homeostasis. The laparoscopic Roux-en-Y gastric bypass patients were noted to have an earlier augmented insulin response potentially mediating improved early glycemic control. However, at three months no significant difference was recorded between the two groups with both procedures markedly improving glucose homeostasis.

Key Points

- The long-term complications and late re-operation rates of vertical-banded gastroplasty are significantly better than those of adjustable silicone gastric banding.
- Improved glucose homeostasis can be equally well achieved by both laparoscopic Roux-en-Y gastric bypass and laparoscopic sleeve gastrectomy.

COLORECTAL

Studies like the MRC CLASSIC trial have helped to establish the role of laparoscopic-assisted surgery for cancer of the colon.[24] The laparoscopic treatment of rectal cancer has however remained controversial. A recently published randomized clinical trial has compared the surgical outcomes of 204 patients after laparoscopic and open approaches for mid and low rectal cancers.[25] Most patients had stage II or III disease and received neo-adjuvant chemoradiation. Sphincter preserving surgery was performed in 79% of patients in the open group and 76% of patients in the laparo-scopic group. Blood loss was significantly greater in the open group (p = <0.001) and operating time was significantly greater in the laparoscopic group (p = 0.020). A return to diet and hospital stay was longer in the open group. Complication rates, involvement of circumferential and radial margins were similar for both procedures. The mean number of isolated lymph nodes was 13.6 in the laparoscopic group compared with 11.6 in the open group (p = 0.026). There were no diffe-rences in local recurrence, disease-free or overall survival.

Key Point

- Laparoscopic surgery for rectal cancer has a similar complication rate to open surgery. It is associated with less blood loss and a shorter hospital stay without compromise of oncological outcome.

The role of radiotherapy in operable rectal cancer has been addressed following the establishment of laparoscopic surgery in this area. A multicenter randomized trial, involving 1350 patients, has compared short course preoperative radiotherapy (25 Gy in 5 fractions) to initial surgery with selective postoperative chemoradiotherapy (45 Gy in 25 fractions with concurrent 5-fluorouracil) restricted to patients with involvement of the circumferential resection margin.[26] At the time of analysis 330 patients had died, 157 in the preoperative radiotherapy group vs 173 in the selective postoperative chemoradiotherapy group. The median follow-up of the surviving patients was four years. During this time 99 patients developed local recurrence, 27 in the preoperative radiotherapy group and 72 in the selective postoperative chemoradiotherapy group. The preoperative radiotherapy group therefore had a 61% reduction in relative risk ($p < 0.001$) and an absolute difference at 3 years of 6.2%. A relative improvement in disease-free survival of 24% (HR 0.76, $p = 0.013$) was recorded in the preoperative radiotherapy group and an absolute difference at 3 years of 6%. Overall survival did not differ between the two groups.

Key Point

- Short-course, pre-operative radiotherapy is an effective treatment for patients with operable colorectal cancer.

Improvements in the medical management of inflammatory bowel disease have reduced the incidence of surgical intervention. However, there are some patients who still require bowel resection. The terminal ileum is the most frequently affected area of the bowel in patients with Crohn's disease. A recently published study with 139 patients has compared recurrence of Crohn's disease following ileocolic stapled side-to-side anastomosis with handsewn anastomosis.[27] Colonoscopy was performed 12 months after surgery. The endoscopic recurrence rate was 42% in the handsewn group compared to 38% in the stapled group ($p = 0.55$). The symptomatic recurrence rate was also comparable, 22% in the handsewn patients compared with 23% in the stapled group ($p = 0.92$). The multivariate logistic regression analysis demonstrated that previous resections were predictive of a higher risk of both endoscopic and symptomatic recurrence. Compliance with postoperative maintenance therapy was predictive of a lower risk of symptomatic recurrence.

Key Point

- The endoscopic and symptomatic recurrence rates after ileocolic resection for Crohn's disease are similar whether a hand sewn end-to-end anastomosis or a stapled side-to-side anastomosis is used.

BREAST SURGERY

Endocrine Treatment

The use of endocrine treatment in breast cancer continues to evolve as alternative therapeutic agents, are developed and the indications for existing drugs are broadened. Compared with tamoxifen, the aromatase inhibitor letrozole improves disease-free survival among postmenopausal women with receptor positive early breast cancer. A phase III randomized double blind trial looked at whether sequential treatment with tamoxifen and letrozole is superior to letrozole alone.[28] Postmenopausal women with hormone receptor positive breast cancer were randomly assigned to receive five years of tamoxifen or letrozole monotherapy or two years of treatment with one agent followed by three years of treatment with the other. At a median follow-up of 71 months disease-free survival was not significantly improved with either sequential treatment as compared with letrozole alone (HR for tamoxifen followed by letrozole 1.05 and for letrozole followed by tamoxifen 0.96). There were more early relapses in women treated with tamoxifen followed by letrozole than among those who received letrozole monotherapy. The difference in overall survival with letrozole monotherapy and tamoxifen monotherapy was not significant.

Key Point

- Letrozole improves disease-free survival in postmenopausal women with endocrine-responsive early breast cancer. There is no advantage in using a switch protocol with tamoxifen.

Radiotherapy

The adjuvant use of radiotherapy, following breast conserving surgery for invasive breast cancer was established following studies, which demonstrated that it reduced the risk of ipsilateral recurrence. Ductal carcinoma *in situ* (DCIS) is a pre-invasive lesion. Follow-up of affected patients has demonstrated that ipsilateral recurrence may be either DCIS or invasive disease. A systematic review of the results of trials investigating the addition of adjuvant radiotherapy to breast conserving surgery for DCIS[29] identified four randomized clinical trials involving 3,925 women. Analysis confirmed a statistically significant benefit from the addition of radiotherapy on all ipsilateral breast events (HR = 0.49, $p < 0.00001$) and ipsilateral DCIS recurrence[30] (HR = 0.64, $p = 0.05$). All subgroups analyzed, including margin status, age and grade benefited from the addition of radiotherapy. Nine women require treatment with radiotherapy to prevent one ipsilateral breast recurrence (NNT = 9). Deaths due to vascular disease, pulmonary toxicity and second cancers were low and not significantly higher in women who received radiotherapy.

Key Point

- The addition of adjuvant radiotherapy to the management of patients treated for DCIS with breast conserving surgery significantly reduces the risk of ipsilateral breast events and recurrence of DCIS. No significant long-term toxicity to radiotherapy has been demonstrated.

Lymphoedema

The risk of lymphoedema following axillary surgery is well established. The quoted incidence can be as high as 30% of patients; however, the number of clinically significant cases is recognized to be much lower. The standard advice to women with breast cancer-related lymphoedema has been to avoid lifting heavy weights with the affected arm. This has prevented them from benefiting from regular exercise, which would increase their bone density. This is of particular importance given the number of patients now treated with aromatase inhibitors. A randomized clinical trial of twice weekly progressive weight lifting has addressed this issue in 141 breast cancer survivors with stable lymphoedema of the arm.[31] The proportion of women who had an increase of 5% or more in limb swelling was similar in the weight-lifting (11%) and the control group (12%). The weight lifting group had greater improvements in self reported severity of lymphoedema symptoms ($p = 0.03$) and a lower incidence of lymphedema exacerbations as assessed by a certified lymphoedema specialist ($p = 0.04$). Upper and lower body strength also improved ($p < 0.001$), compared with the control group. There were no reported adverse events related to the intervention.

Key Point

- Breast cancer patients with upper limb lymphoedema who follow a program of slow progressive weight lifting have a decreased incidence of exacerbations of lymphoedema, reduced symptoms and increased strength.

REFERENCES

1. Paochroen V, Mingmalairak C, Apisarnthanarak A. Comparison of surgical wound infection after pre-operative skin preparation with 4% chlorhexidine and providone iodine: a prospective randomized trial. Journal of the Medical Association of Thailand 2009;92(7):898-902.
2. Franczyk M, Lohman RF, Agarwal JP, Rupani G, Drum M, Gottlieb LJ. The impact of topical lidocaine on pain level assessment during and after vacuum-assisted closure dressing changes: a double-blind, prospective ramdomized study. Plastic and Reconstructive Surgery 2009;124(3):854-61.
3. O'Malley GF, Dominici P, Giraldo P, Aguilera E, Verma M, Lares C, et al. Routine packing of simple cutaneous abscesses is painful and probably unnecessary. Academic Emergency Medicine 2009;16(5):470-3.

4. Kerger KH, Mascha E, Steinbrecher B, Frietsch T, Radke OC, Stoecklein K, et al. Routine use of nasogastric tubes does not reduce postoperative nausea and vomiting. Anesthsia and Analgesia 2009;109:768-73.

5. Appukutty J, Shroff PP. Nasogastric tube insertion using different techniques in anesthetized patients: a prospective randomised study. Anesthsia and Analgesia 2009;109(3):832-5.

6. Halm JA, Lip H, Schmitz PL, Jeekel J. Incisional hernia after upper abdominal surgery: a randomized controlled trial of midline versus transverse incision. Hernia 2009;13(3):275-80.

7. Forbes SS, Eskicioglu C, McLeod RS, Okrainec A. Meta-analysis of randomized controlled trials comparing open and laparoscopic ventral and incisional hernia repair with mesh. British Journal of Surgery 2009;96(8):851-8.

8. Taha AS, McCloskey C, Prasad R, Bezlyak V. Famotidine for the prevention of peptic ulcers and oesophagitis in patients taking low-dose aspirin (FAMOUS): a phase III, randomized, double-blind, placebo-controlled trial Lancet 2009;374(9684):119-25.

9. Javid G, Zargar SA, U-Saif R, Khan BA, Yatoo GN, Shah AH, et al. Comparison of poor IV proton pump inhibitors on 72-hour intragastric pH in bleeding peptic ulcer. Journal Gastroenterolgy and Hepatology 2009; 24(7):1236-43.

10. Bertleff MJ, Halm JA, Bemelman WA, van der Ham AC, van der Harst E, Oei HI, et al. Randomized clinical trial of laparoscopic versus open repair of the perforated peptic ulcer: the LAMA Trial. World Journal of Surgery 2009;33(7):1368-73.

11. Shaheen NJ, Sharma P, Overholt BF, et al. Radiofrequency ablation in Barrett's esophagus with dysplasia. New England Journal of Medicine 2009; 360(22):2277-88.

12. Hall NJ, Pacilli M, Eaton S, et al. Recovery after open versus laparoscopic pyloromyotomy for pyloric stenosis: a double-blind multicentre randomized controlled trial. Lancet 2009;373(9661):390-8.

13. Abid S, Jafri W, Hamid S, et al. Terlipressin vs octreotide in bleeding oesophageal varices as an adjunct therapy with endoscopic and ligation: a randomized double blind placebo-controlled trial. The American Journal of Gastroenterology 2009;104(3):617-23.

14. Orloff MJ, Isenberg JI, Wheeler HO, et al. Randomized Trial of Emergency Endoscopic Sclerotherapy Versus Emergency Portacaval Shunt for Acutely Bleeding Eosophageal Varices in Cirrhosis. Journal of the American College of Surgeons 2009;209(1):25-40.

15. Amin MA, El-Gendy MM, Dawoud IE, et al. Partial splenic embolisation versus splenectomy for the management of hypersplenism in cirrhotic patients. World Journal of Surgery 2009;33(8):1702-10.

16. Ruers TJ, Wiering B, van der Sijp JR, et al. Improved selection of patients for hepatic surgery of colorectal liver metastases with (18)F-FDG PET: a randomized study. The Journal of Nuclear Medicine 2009;50(7):1036-41.

17. Olah A, Issekutz A, Belagyi T, et al. Randomized clinical trial of techniques for closure of the pancreatic remnant following distal pancreatectomy. British Journal of Surgery 2009;96(6):602-7.

18. Ueno H, Kosuge T, Matsuyama Y, et al. A randomized phase III trial comparing gemcitabine with surgery-only in patients with resected

pancreatic cancer: Japanese Study Group of Adjuvant Therapy for Pancreatic Cancer. British Journal of Cancer 2009;101(6):908-15.

19. Petrov MS, Savides TJ. Systematic review of endoscopic ultrasonography versus endoscopic retrograde cholangiopancreatography for suspected choledocholithiasis. British Journal of Surgery 2009;96(9):967-74.

20. Bai Y, Xu C, Yang X, et al. Glyceryl trinitrate for prevention of pancreatitis after endoscopic retrograde cholangiopancreatography: a meta-analysis of randomized, double-blind, placebo-controlled trials. Endoscopy 2009;41(8):690-5.

21. Cennamo V, Fuccio L, Zagari RM, et al. Can a wire-guided cannulation technique increase bile duct cannulation rate and prevent post-ERCP pancreatitis?: A meta-analysis of randomized controlled trials. The American Journal of Gastroenterology 2009;104(9):2343-50.

22. Scozzari G, Farinella E, Bonnet G, et al. Laparoscopic adjustable silicone gastric banding vs laparoscopic vertical banded gastroplasty in morbidly obese patients: long-term results of a prospective randomized controlled clinical trial. Obesity Surgery 2009;19(8):1108-15.

23. Peterli R, Wolnerhassen B, Peters T, et al. Improvement in glucose metabolism after bariatric surgery: comparison of laparoscopic Roux-en-Y gastric bypass and laparoscopic sleeve gastrectomy: a prospective randomized trial. Annals of Surgery 2009;250(2):234-41.

24. Guillou P, Quirke H, Thorpe J, et al. Short-term endpoints of conventional versus laparoscopic-assisted surgery in patients with colorectal cancer (MRC CLASSIC trial): multicentre, randomized controlled trial. Lancet 2005; 365(9472):1718-26.

25. Lujan J, Valero G, Hernandez Q, et al. Randomized clinical trial comparing laparoscopic and open surgery in patients with rectal cancer. British Journal of Surgery 2009;96(9):982-9.

26. Sebag-Montefiore D, Stephens RJ, Steele R, et al. Preoperative radiotherapy versus selective postoperative chemoradiotherapy in patients with rectal cancer (MRC CR07 and NCIC-CTG C016): a multicentre, randomized trial. Lancet 2009;373(9666):811-20.

27. McLeod RS, Wolff BG, Ross S, et al. Recurrence of Crohn's disease after ileocolic resection is not affected by anastomotic type: results of a multicentre, randomized controlled trial. Diseases of the Colon and Rectum 2009;52(5):919-27.

28. The BIG1-98 Colloaborative Group Letrozole therapy alone or in sequence with tamoxifen in women with breast cancer. New England Journal of Medicine 2009;361(8):766-76.

29. Goodwin A, Parker S, Ghersi D, Wilcken N. Post-operative radiotherapy for ductal carcinoma in situ of the breast- a systematic review of the randomized trials. Breast 2009;18(3):143-9.

30. Goodwin A, Parker S, Ghersi D, Wilcken N. Post-operative radiotherapy for ductal carcinoma in situ of the breast. Cochrane Database Systematic Review 2009;8(3):CD000563

31. Schmitz KH, Ahmen RL, Troxel A, et al. Weight lifting in women with breast-cancer-related lymphoedema. New England Journal of Medicine 2009; 361(7):664-73.

Index

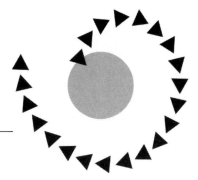

235